# ANCIENT TRAVELS

Cover design by Matthew Rayback
Cover art by Iva Lim Peck, L.Ac.
Chinese translation on the cover by Jen Sin Lau of Singapore

Chinese paintings (pp. 12, 30, 70, 82, 100, 128, 140, 146, 156, 186, 190, 204, 256, 288) by Iva Lim Peck , L.Ac., 1979–1981
Bamboo paintings (pp. 220, 272, 276, 286) by Richard A. Peck, L.Ac., 1976–1979

Distributed by
P & R Medical Services, Inc.
P. O. Box 262488
Plano, TX 75026
www.AncientTravels.com

This book is a work of fiction. It is not intended for use in the actual treatment of patients. Any similarity between the book's characters or events with real people or events is purely coincidental.

ISBN: 144143920X
EAN-13: 9781441439208

# ANCIENT TRAVELS

A Discourse Between a Master and His Student on
Acupuncture and Chinese Martial Arts

Richard A. Peck, L.Ac.

With Illustrations by Iva Lim Peck, L.Ac.

# CONTENTS

# EXCERPTS

Chapter 2, page 14—"How is it, thought Liu, looking at the tree again and its lesson, that the wisdom of nature, without a consciousness, can be transmitted to us humans?"

Chapter 6, page 75—"It appears you have a condition referred to as Liver Fire Rising."

Chapter 7, page 91—"Your problem is multi-faceted. I will try to take care of you, but to answer your question, all health care issues can be simplified to an imbalance of Yin and Yang."

Chapter 7, page 93—"Pregnancy should be a time of joy and happiness and not a time of sickness."

Chapter 11, page 129—"Actually, practicing Tai Chi Chuan will go a long way in reducing or preventing arthritis, high blood pressure, strokes, and heart attacks."

Chapter 13, page 145—"At first, I felt nothing, but now I feel this overall warming of my right shoulder and the pain is going away."

Chapter 14, page 150—"No, Pei Ke. These men are here to kill me. Unfortunately, you are here and they have decided your fate. Do exactly as I say."

Chapter 15, page 157—"Today Pei Ke had his palms facing downward as if he were trying to make a connection with the center of the earth."

Chapter 18, page 178—"The third failing is the lack of understanding about the four diagnostic procedures. This is because the doctor does not have a full grasp of the concepts of Yin and Yang and the theory of Five Elements."

Chapter 21, page 199—"This technique increases the amount of Qi along the Conception Vessel Meridian and tonifies the energy. It will substantially help her incontinence."

.

# PREFACE

This book will appeal to a wide range of readers. If your interest is Chinese culture, you will find the story and its content educational. Even though it is a work of fiction, I have endeavored to make the setting and information as accurate as possible.

If you are learning Oriental Medicine or are a patient (or potential patient) of Oriental Medicine, you may find this book helpful in understanding the diverse and difficult concepts of this four thousand year old art. I hope this book will help you understand that there are other avenues to your health care.

If you are a practitioner of Oriental Medicine, this book will help you explain to your patients why you are doing what you are doing, and the desired results of your treatment process. The explanations in the book are simple enough for nearly everyone to understand, but comprehensive enough to help nonprofessionals gain an understanding of the subject.

My sincere thanks go to my first teachers, Huo Chi Kwang, Dr. Ineon Moon, Master Lu Hung Bin, and Dr. Tsao Cheng Chang for pointing the way on this path of martial arts and Oriental Medicine. I treasure their continuous encouragement in those early days of studying, especially when everything seemed to be overwhelming. I feel blessed.

I would also like to thank Dr. Devi Nambudripad, Dr. Tae-Woo Yoo, Dr. Ming Qing Zhu, and Dr. Richard Tan who willingly shared their expertise helping me to increase and mature in my ability to treat patients.

Thanks go to Mat. Rayback, Sally Kemp, Jeremy Freeman, Patsy Keyser, Landa Miller, Victor Yannacone, Carol Yannacone, Dr. Mark Hanson, Dr. Jake Green, Don Jones, Mike Sherrod, Bill Skelton, Tim Franz, Jack Howe, Kent Williamson, Linda Donahue, Julia Mandala, Barbara Baker, John E. Peck, my son David A. Peck and my wife Iva Lim Peck for reading the manuscript and giving their valuable insight into how to make this novel more accurate and readable.

Most of all my appreciation goes to the many students and patients who, over the years of my practice of Oriental Medicine, unknowingly taught me so much about how to be a better teacher and practitioner. I owe them a debt of gratitude. Without them, this book would not be possible.

My thanks to my wife Iva Lim Peck who allowed me to use her paintings. I hope you will enjoy the book. Any errors or emissions are strictly my own doing. If you feel there is an error in the book please bring this to my attention. Please e-mail your comments or suggestions for inclusion in my next book.

Note that the surnames of Liu and Pei are commonly used in China. Liu Bin and Pei Ke are the main characters in this novel. This is entirely a work of fiction and there is no connection or similarity between its characters, places, events, and anyone in the past, present, or future.

Richard A. Peck, L.Ac. (September 2009)
www.AncientTravels.com
www.IntegratedCenterForOrientalMedicine.com

# PROLOGUE

The first cool wind of autumn blew over the remote mountains of Northern China, bringing with it a blast of arctic air that was a harbinger of what was still to come in that fateful autumn. In a few, short weeks, the snow would fall, forming snowdrifts so deep and impassable that the valley would be shut off to all but the hardiest of travelers.

Only a few paths led through the mountains and these were dangerous. Few dared to be caught where shelter or food was nonexistent, and travelers who were unaware of the correct route usually perished.

Those hardy ones who did make it into the valley were awestruck by its natural beauty. In the early spring, lush from the runoff of melting snow, it became a paradise. The same runoff, along with rain directed at higher elevations by the natural contours of the land, carved natural streams into the landscape, and the moisture flowed downward to form a cold, deep lake filled with fish.

The shape of the land, gently sloped from mountains to valley, lent itself to a limited cultivation of rice. Enough flat land existed on the downward slope that the people could have three small rice fields. The runoff from one terraced rice paddy fed the paddy below. Wheat grew and farm animals grazed in the remaining areas. The valley was perfect for those who wanted to be self-sufficient, away from outsiders, but still within a half-day's journey to a nearby settlement.

In this remote land, the first member of the Liu family, Liu Ma Hao, had staked his claim to the land, many generations before. His claim was not without controversy and strife, for many other families also claimed the land. Liu Ma Hao, however, had influence with the reigning emperor and the wealthy so the land became his. Still, the locals' concern about the land's rightful owners lingered for decades.

Stories among those who felt displaced, forgotten, or unjustly omitted in the distribution of the land predicted that one day this land and its wealthy harvest would return to its rightful owners, whether by force or by other means.

As these prophecies festered, the Liu family insured that the land and the surrounding people were in harmony with each other and with the Tao. The Tao, according to Chinese philosophy, kept the order and balance of things.

The Tao (or Way) was responsible for every interaction, from the rising of the sun to the changes of life. Taoism along with Confucianism and Buddhism were the moral threads that held society together. These three philosophical beliefs developed independently. Though each had its own unique structure, they blended into one thought pattern.

The all-encompassing Tao held the positive and negative forces of nature in check. Buddhism gave the people their beliefs and a form of worship, while Confucianism held the moral order together. No matter the power of this collection of Chinese thought, greed, jealousy, and human frailties constantly threatened this underlying Chinese thought pattern. Greed and jealously often led to revenge. Eventually, greed, jealously, and revenge led to unspeakable crimes.

# CHAPTER ONE

It would be another two hours before the sun rose on this cool autumn morning. In the temple where he lived, Liu Bin, a son of the Liu family, usually woke quietly and peacefully, but today he felt an unsettling in his heart. He had felt this apprehension before and knew it indicated turmoil and conflict within the Universal Tao.

As he had matured in body and spirit, he had also matured in the wisdom of the Way. Thus he knew that the manner in which the resolution of conflict took place was the only important factor. In this case, he sensed his pending involvement, whether or not he wanted it. He was not fond of these resolutions, but the forces of nature were too strong to fight. It was better to go along with the flow, for the flow agreed with the Taoist philosophy of peacefulness, balance, and internal harmony.

He arose quickly from his sleeping area in the temple. He changed from his nightclothes into his martial arts attire and headed for the path to his training area. He had taken this route next to the creek and through the bamboo forest daily for the last ten years.

As Liu walked away from the main gate, he first came to the Happy Panda Spring. The spring provided water for the temple inhabitants. It could not be seen unless one knew where to look: behind the path in a slight clearing among the dense foliage. Years earlier, the monks had purposely concealed the clearing to give the area a sense of tranquility.

Happy Panda Spring had been named for one of the monks who had previously lived at the temple. The monk enjoyed the solitude of the spring so much that he built the stonework and seating area that partially surrounded it. The sound of trickling water and the chirping of birds had brought continuous joy to those who meditated under the tall bamboo trees.

Often, when Liu came to this spot to sit and meditate, he thought of the monk who had long since departed into heavenly bliss. Liu had heard stories about the day the monk did not return from his meditation. When the other monks arrived at his meditating spot, all they found were his clothes neatly folded and placed on his favorite rock. Since there were no signs of struggle, they assumed he had finally found the means to enter into everlasting life.

A short distance beyond the spring, the path rose abruptly, wound up towards the mountain, and opened around the rim of a precipice. Liu enjoyed this twenty-minute walk and the contrast between the claustrophobia of the bamboo forest below and the openness of the mountain above. It was similar to the Yin and Yang, an aspect of the underlying driving force that controlled the actions of nature—a force which he was committed to serve and which he knew would serve him in return.

Each time he walked along the edge, he knew that one false step would tumble him hundreds of feet to his death, but as always, his training held true. Each step was soft and agile, yet the placement of his foot was rooted, firmly connected to the Yin energy of the earth. Before the commitment to the earth was made, however, he could withdraw his foot at the slightest lack of firmness in the Yin energy. No matter how dark it was, he relied on this insight.

This era was the Qing Dynasty, which lasted from 1644 until 1911 when the last emperor, Pu Yi was overthrown in the great revolution. This was also a time of great tragedy for many Chinese people. The importation of opium ruined millions of lives and families. Originally, the opium came from India in trade for tea and silk that the British imported.

After many years, the Chinese government banned its importation. In the 1830's, ten million people were addicted to opium. Government crack down on the importation of opium led to two opium wars. The Chinese, with their small coastal navy, succumbed to the far superior British warships and armed merchant vessels. The Treaty of Nanking followed the Chinese defeat; as a result, Hong Kong was thus ceded to the British. The importation of opium, however, continued to be a problem. Growing up as a child, Liu was neither aware of nor touched by the opium, as he lived with his family in modest comfort far from the influence of foreigners.

Liu Bin was born in the year of the monkey and was the second son of Liu Chang. The celestial animals and their designations developed from antiquity and appeared in various aspects of Chinese culture. Of the twelve celestial animals—rat, ox, tiger, hare, dragon, snake, horse, sheep, monkey, rooster, dog, and boar—the celestial monkey above all others was considered intelligent, creative, intuitive, and happy.

Except for his father, he was the only one in his family who walked the enlightened path of the Taoist tradition. His sister, bound by tradition was promised to another family where she would continue their bloodline. His older brother, Liu Ming, fulfilled the ancient tradition of providing a male heir to carry on the family name. His two younger twin brothers were more inclined towards the finer things in life and accordingly had been somewhat pampered while their mother was alive.

As a boy, Liu learned to read and write from his mother and paternal grandmother. They also taught him painting, calligraphy, and poetry, all of which influenced his future life.

At the same time, his father began shaping his body. A powerful man, he wanted all his sons to carry on the martial arts tradition of the family. When Liu Bin was six, his father began teaching him strength-building exercises. The training began with sit-ups and leg bends. It progressed to horse stances where he stood with feet parallel and shoulder width apart in a half-sitting position, his palms together in front of his face.

As he developed strength, Liu learned additional flexibility routines originating from the Buddhist martial art of Shaolin. His training at home continued until he was twenty. Later, he learned the Taoist martial arts of Tai Chi Chuan, Hsing-Yi Chuan, and Pa Kua Chang. These arts were matched equally with his later training in healing and Qi cultivation. His father, his paternal grandfather, and his great grandfather before him, had each produced at least one male offspring to carry on the secrets of the family tradition. Liu alone chose, in a time of inner turmoil, to seek out others who could help him take his training past the boundaries of those family members before him. He forsook family life, its pleasures, rewards, and hardships and entered a realm none of his ancestors had traveled before.

What would he do with what he had accomplished? This thought bothered him on this day as he approached the autumn of his life. At his age, time had the advantage, but soon he must face reality and put aside his idealism.

His personal training area, for he alone had use of the space, was to the left of the path many feet from the mountain's edge. He had an unobstructed view of the distant valley. It was significant that his secluded place looked out on the rising sun. He had been taught to face East in the mornings when doing Qi Gong, and not North as those he saw in the countryside. The rising sun provided one aspect of the Yang energy just as the moon in the evening provided one aspect of the Yin energy. A new day always brought the invigoration of new energy.

From his vantage point, he saw where generations of farmers had struggled to survive. The land, terraced in all directions, took advantage of the water descending from the very tops of the surrounding mountains. Each terrace captured the water before it passed on to the next lower terrace. The water and silt from the mountainside eventually flowed into streams that ultimately formed a river. In turn, the river would take the water and the silt hundreds of miles to another group of farmers who depended on the yearly flooding to rejuvenate their land.

"How similar we humans are to this process," thought Liu. "Both our lives and the lives of the plants around us are dependant on water. Our lives and nature are intrinsically meshed, each a small part of the whole Taoist picture."

The slight, almost imperceptible rustling of fallen leaves immediately attracted Liu's attention. He had long ago learned to listen, as others had not, and to see as others did not see. The emerging figure was the last student he was to take.

"Good morning, Master," Pei Ke said.

"Good morning," said Liu Bin. "The sun will be rising shortly. Let us begin."

Qi Gong exercises were the foundation of all Chinese internal martial arts. Not only did these exercises build strong leg and back muscles, they also increased flexibility and sensitivity.

The basic exercises he had taught Pei Ke were a compilation of Qi Gong exercises he had learned from his father, who had learned them from those who had walked the enlightened path. Liu treasured these exercises. They built within him a tremendous amount of internal energy that he could focus and control at will to use for healing or self-defense.

Liu firmly believed that to be a good martial artist, one needed to be a good healer, and to be a good healer, one needed to be a good martial artist. They mirrored the concept of Yin and Yang. Liu had seen many martial artists who taught Qi Gong, but had no knowledge of the healing arts. These martial artists were unable to explain to their students the concepts of Qi Gong. He had also known many healers who had depleted their own energy in the process of healing others. They lacked the knowledge of developing the universal energy within themselves.

Pei Ke had been studying from Liu for two years. He was not unusually bright, but had those qualities every teacher looks for in a student. He was dedicated, loyal, and learned quickly. What he lacked in one attribute he made up for in another.

Maybe it is true, thought Liu. Not only does the student seek the enlightened teacher, but the teacher waits for that one student who will accept his teachings and pass those teachings onto the next generation. Since Liu had no son, he had chosen Pei Ke to join a few others who had committed to carry on this tradition.

Still, Pei Ke was different. Liu had taught others before, but their earthly commitments, with their pleasures and responsibilities, always hampered their learning. Many had learned but few had left with an adequate understanding of the arts he taught. The majority of those he had taught had only learned one of the internal martial arts, and in most cases had left with only a cursory understanding of the art. No one but Pei Ke and a few others had the dedication, drive, stamina, and willingness to put up with the hardships.

Liu remembered the many hours of training he had endured during his lifetime. In the early years, he was made to squat in the horse stance for as long as he could. Initially, he could do it for only a few moments. As time passed, however, he was able to maintain it indefinitely. Later when he studied Pa Kua Chang, he learned to walk the circle. He did this for an extended period of time, gradually lowering the levels of sitting while his teacher continuously corrected his posture. The result of this and other training was his incredibly strong legs.

He was taught that developing strong legs was the foundation of rooting oneself to the ground. It helped one meditate and develop internal Qi. Many times as he was practicing an exceptionally low position, his teachers would have him hold it for extended periods of time. A gentle but firm hand on his shoulder would prevent him from rising. Usually a lengthy lecture would ensue that would take his mind off the pain.

"Master," Pei Ke said. "You always time our exercises so that when we hold the universal ball, the sun starts to rise in the east."

"Haven't you noticed when you are holding the ball, your body is more awake and the rising sun sends warmth through your body that reaches to the core of your essence? This rush of energy prepares you for the remaining exercises, just as the exercises prior to holding the ball prepared you for the energy of the sun."

"Then all the exercises are important."

"Yes, and they should be done in the order I have taught them. Each of the fourteen exercises accomplishes something different and the whole is greater than the sum of the individual parts."

Liu paused, then added, "However, if the vicissitudes of life descend on you, and you do not have time to do all the exercises, the most important is holding the universal ball, for it is the gathering of the energy of the awakening day."

"I know you have demonstrated numerous times the correct posture for holding the ball. Why is this so critical?"

"The energy that surrounds us is there for all to take. It is the universal energy. It came before the beginning of time and it will be here long after we leave. Our bodies are an accumulation of it. We are an embodiment of what came before us. When you practice holding the Tai Chi ball, you must do it correctly so your body and its energy can tap into the universal energy."

"Show me?" Pei Ke said.

Liu nodded and positioned himself so his weight was centered on his back foot, while the heel of his forward foot was raised slightly. He turned his waist approximately forty-five degrees, then turned his head to watch as his student tried to imitate the position.

"Lift the heel of your forward foot."

"Why?" Pei Ke said. He did as he was instructed, though.

"You must stimulate the Yong Quan point," Liu answered. "It is the beginning of the energy pathway that runs along the inside of the leg and enters into the kidneys. Doctors call it the Kidney Meridian and it is the main essence of the energy source that keeps us alive. It feels warm, even tingly."

"But Master, how does raising my forward foot stimulate this pathway?"

"The energy of the universe comes to us in many different ways. Sometimes it is linear and sometimes circular. When the energy is powerful, it feels like a wave or a pulsing sensation. Often, for those with internal disharmony, the energy is scattered. You want to tap into both the linear energy and the circular or spiraling energy. When the Yong Quan acupuncture point on the forward foot is lined up with the acupuncture points Yin Tang, Qi Hai, and Shan Zhong, your body will be in linear alignment. This linear alignment gives the body its structural integrity. When done correctly, the position is almost effortless."

He looked back toward the rising sun and lifted his arms to continue.

"Now," he said, "place your arms at chest height with the palms facing towards your chest. Now draw an imaginary line from the Lao Gong acupuncture point on center of each palm to the Shan Zhong point on the center of your chest. A triangle will be formed."

"Why is such precision necessary?" Pei Ke said.

"Remember, I mentioned to you that the martial art of Pa Kua Chang is circular in its motions and applications. It is believed by some that the circles of Pa Kua Chang are nothing more than a series of very small continuously formed angles. The structural integrity of Pa Kua Chang comes from the angles, and the structural integrity of holding the ball helps to develop the internal energy."

"Am I doing it correctly?" He looked eager.

"No," Liu said, ignoring the boy's look of disappointment. "Your thumbs must be raised slightly and the fingers separated with the middle fingers bent slightly toward you to stimulate the energy of the Pericardium Meridian. Hold your hands so that only a few inches separate your middle fingers. The small space between the hands must intersect the imaginary line running from the Lao Gong point to Yin Tang point between your eyebrows. When you succeed in doing this correctly, you will tap into the universal energy."

"Yes Master," Pei Ke said, trying to sound serene. "I now feel a warmth and a tingling sensation throughout my body."

"Good. Then tell me how you should position your body to align its structure and open the energy flows within? Trying to assimilate the universal energy when the gates of the body are closed only hampers and frustrates the learning process."

Pei Ke thought for a moment, then answered, shifted his body as he did to demonstrate his words.

"My shoulders are slightly forward and my pelvis is tucked in," he said. "And my head should be erect, but how do I make sure it is in the right position?"

"You have forgotten?"

"No, Master. It is always interesting for you to explain it again. Each time you explain these concepts my understanding is enhanced."

"I have told you this before," Liu said. "You must pay better attention. Now, draw an imaginary line from the bottom of your earlobe to the top of your ear and up to the top of your head. Then imagine another line from the tip of your nose over the highest part of your head. Where these two lines intersect is the meeting point of the energy of your whole body. This is one of the entry points for the universal life force. Now you want to hold your head so that you can visualize a connection between this point and the farthest reaches of the heavens.

"The ancients referred to this acupuncture point as Bai Hui, the meeting point of the energy and it is the point where all Yang energy meets. Since Yang energy and Yin energy are complementary and one flows into the other, this point is important in the overall scheme of meditation. It is often used to treat headaches, hemorrhoids, and back pain. Very skilled doctors use this point to treat mental and emotional problems. In addition, there are points one inch above, below, and to the left and right of Bai Hui that can be used to help those with poor memory.

"Now, imagine a slight tug on this point and try to feel the upward pulling of the skin on your face and neck. Your chin should drop slightly and your head will become erect. In the process, the neck will open up and allow the energy to flow correctly through your body.

Remember, that when the head is lifted up, there is a tendency to look down as the chin drops. Do not look downward, rather look straight ahead and you will feel a little pressure between your eyebrows. This will stimulate the third eye area. Do you understand?"

"Yes, Master. Is this correct?"

Liu sighed.

"Your head is correct, but you have moved your shoulders. Here. Put your hand on my upper back, on the space between the spine and the scapular. Observe what happens when I move my shoulders forward: both scapulars move away from the spine. This motion and deep breathing allows the chest to become hollow."

"Master..."

"Enough questions for one day. Just follow along with me as I complete the fourteen exercises. The sun is now up and we have missed the opportunity for the day."

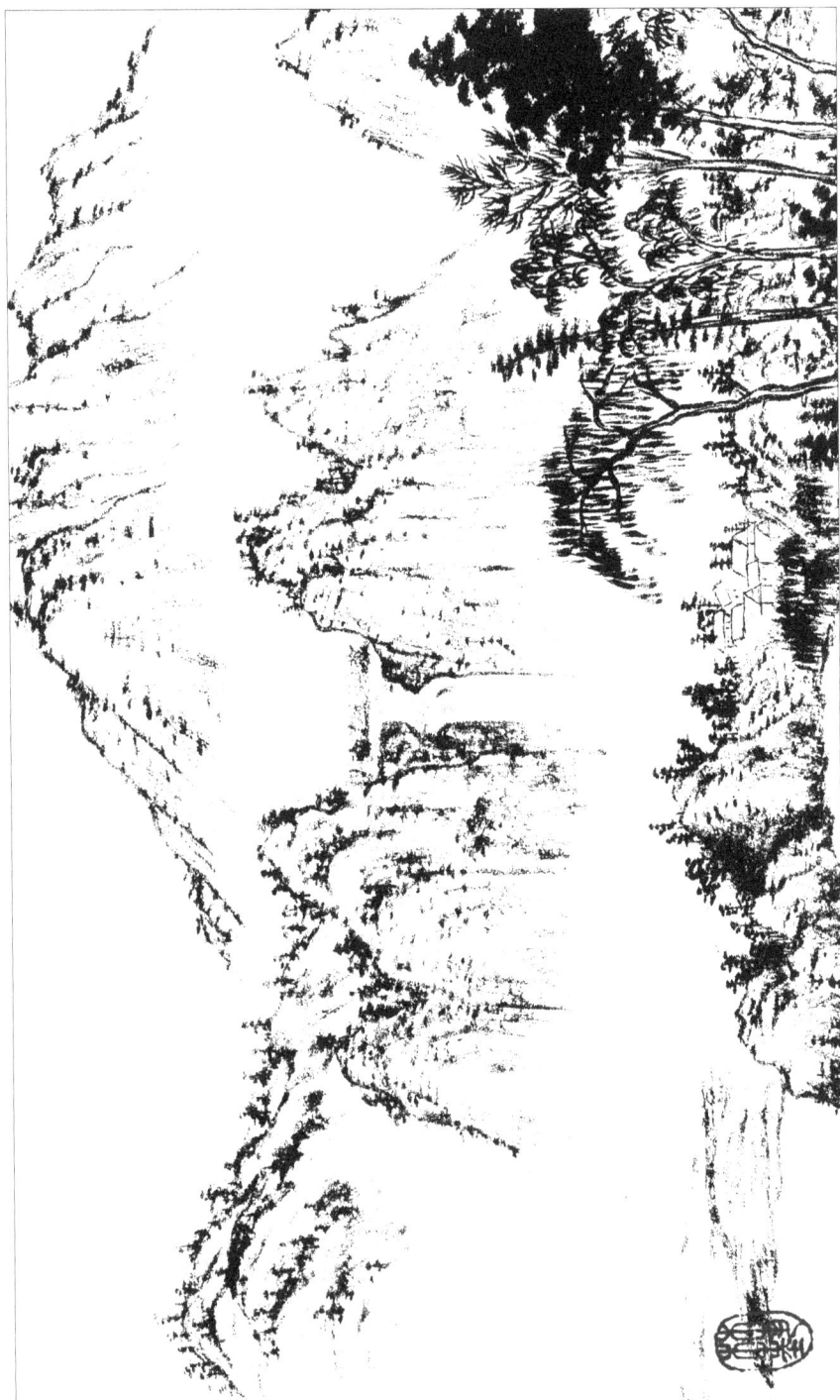

# Chapter Two

Pei Ke and Liu Bin walked slowly back to the temple. Liu had spent a good part of the morning teaching Pei Ke. As the boy practiced, Liu meditated. Liu had learned the external or "Wai Dan" method of meditation first from his grandfather and then from his father. As he progressed in age and maturity his father taught those internal arts referred to as "Nei Dan."

Although the foundation for his martial arts came from his family, it was his extensive travels throughout China, an inquisitive nature, and his studies with some of the great internal martial art masters that allowed him to develop his internal energy. This energy defined him not only physically but also mentally and spiritually.

What would he do with Pei Ke? He appeared to be a good student, but asked too many questions. Maybe the questions were his way of learning. Maybe the questions would speed up the learning process. Would Pei Ke be willing to make the sacrifice that Liu willingly made so long ago? Would Pei Ke shun the excesses of the world and dedicate himself to a monastic life?

As the master and student approached the temple they passed a gnarled old tree. Liu had watched the woodcutters come many times over the years to cut trees, but they always bypassed this crooked tree in favor of the beautiful trees nearby. The old tree, which grew among big rocks, struggled just to exist, whereas the ones less rooted were the ones the woodcutters favored. The complex root system of the old tree had given it its long life and it made Liu think of his father, who had taught him that the ability to root the body to the Yin energy of the earth would enhance his martial arts, meditation, and longevity. Not for the first time, he wondered what his father would have done had he been faced with the concerns that faced Liu.

How is it, thought Liu, looking at the tree again and its lesson, that the wisdom of nature, without a consciousness, can be transmitted to us humans? Or maybe there is a consciousness within nature. When we become one with the Tao, our spirit will enjoy the fruits of our earthly meditative labors.

Liu's living quarters in the temple were located away from the others, though there was nothing special about them. He had a narrow bed with a straw-filled pad to keep the chill from entering from below. In the winter, a metal pan with heated rocks sat under the bed. He slept on a dried tealeaf pillow. He believed the leaves soothed his mind and warded off the cold from his lungs. The comforter he put over himself was filled with silk, which was extremely warm in the winter months. He eschewed the materials most people used for cover because those materials weighted down the body, giving it fitful sleep.

The seven monks practiced a combination of Taoism and Buddhism. Liu was not a monk but shared with them as they shared with him. A mutual respect and dependency developed among the group. The monks did not try to influence Liu's convictions nor he theirs. In return for the monks' providing his meager room and sharing whatever food was offered by the local inhabitants, Liu treated their health problems and provided a measure of security. Because of his impeccable command of the internal martial arts, his reputation fell somewhere between famous and infamous.

His philosophical beliefs were out of favor, for they combined the teachings of more than one way of life. Because of his diverse training, he followed the road that would later be called a hybrid version of I Quan Tao. It encompassed all things beautiful within the various philosophies and religions of the time, which he blended seamlessly into one concept. Of course, the Buddhists disavowed any association with such a philosophy because it did not follow all the tenants of Buddhist beliefs. So it was for the other major and, for that matter, minor philosophies. None of them accepted Liu's belief or wanted any part of his philosophy. The ruling factions thought Liu dangerous to the way of life of the common man. Those in command feared that the common man had little or no influence as an individual, but was all-powerful when and if united with others like himself. It was necessary to put down, conquer or suppress that which was different. And, so it was with Liu. The monks did him a favor just as he did them a favor. As long as his relationship with the monks did not draw undue attention, it could be continued indefinitely.

Breakfast was like any meal; it depended on the offerings from the local populace. Most often, it consisted of soybean milk, sweetened with a little bit of sugar or honey, and some vegetable filled buns. The monks would never eat meat because they believed life was precious, and one should not kill his fellow man or animal. In fact, they believed everything should be done to preserve life. Even animals had a spiritual essence here on earth that should not be jeopardized. Midday meal was usually a mixed portion of steamed rice, vegetables, or fruits. Whenever possible, the meal was a combination of Yin and Yang, for Yin and Yang existed in everything. If there was a dark-colored vegetable, then there was usually a light-colored vegetable on the same plate, or on another plate.

Yin and Yang was a simple, beautiful, and practical concept that was the underlying philosophy of Taoism. It permeated everything in Chinese thought, work, medicine, martial arts, and life. The Yin represented the negative, dark, withdrawn, slow, female, and emotional aspect. The Yang represented the positive, bright, outward, fast, male, and unemotional aspect. Thus, the Yin is what makes the Yang what it is. The force of the female compliments and makes the male. The darkness of the Yin is not an unfavorable aspect to be scorned or looked down upon, but rather an enhancement of the other. In fact, the Yin is the power of the Tao, the softness overcoming the hardness. The negative aspect of Yin is never associated as being undesirable. For one to say that the darkness, negative, and female characteristics of Yin are bad is only to show a misunderstanding of the Tao. This concept of complimentary opposites is what holds the universe together, and what gave Liu his insight into the workings of not only his immediate surroundings, but also of the world he entered into in meditation.

Meditation is always done either sitting or standing. It could be done lying on one's back if one is sick, but it is never done lying on the abdomen. Like everything in life, there are reasons for the right way and the wrong way. The ancients, through trial and error, discovered that the energy from the universe enters into the body through portals. The portals must be aligned with the linear but spiraling energy coming to us. Sitting, standing, and lying on one's back are the only ways for these portals to open up to accept the universal energy.

"Master Liu, please come quickly."

The Abbott of the temple, Feng Que, was calling him. The Abbott was a small man, but he assumed an outward position of authority. He was the glue holding the temple together and gave the populace the feeling that the temple provided a useful existence. In essence, each monk was a separate entity following his own road of enlightenment. However, as a collective group, they gave a valuable gift of peacefulness, hopefulness, and direction to the community.

"What is the matter?" Liu asked.

"Ma Guang Yah is having difficulty breathing and is asking for you."

Liu rose from his breakfast.

"I will come immediately. Where is he now?"

"Follow me and I will take you to him."

The temple at its inception, and Liu's suggestion, was eight-sided, which conformed to the theory of the I-Ching and the principles of Feng Shui. Its inner walls were circular, resembling the Yin Yang circle while the outside walls were exactly the same distance from the opposite side, thus containing and enhancing the flow of energy within the structure. While the combination of Yin Yang and eight-sided walls did not conform to the design of typical temples, the concept seemed to work for the inhabitants of that temple, for they were all in unity with each other.

"Master?"

"Yes, Pei Ke."

"May I come with you?"

"Yes."

"While we walk to see Ma Guang Yah, may I be so bold as to ask you a few questions?"

"Of course."

"Master, Ma Guang Yah is suffering with his sickness. Why do we have pain and sickness?"

Liu smiled faintly. Pei Ke certainly did not hold back.

"That question has been asked since the first human learned to think for himself. There is no good answer, but maybe this will help in a general way. The energy in our bodies flows in a continuous circular pattern. Disruption of that energy for any reason will cause us to experience health problems. These health problems can be pain, internal sickness, or even emotional problems."

"Then what interferes with the flow of our internal energy?"

"It can be disturbed by either external or internal factors. An external factor could be a severe bruise or injury that blocks the flow of energy at the site of the injury or anywhere along the energy pathway. It could also be a pathogenic factor from the outside affecting the body. Internal factors can be caused by heredity or the food and drink we consume. Each health care issue has signs and symptoms for you to discover. These signs and symptoms can be differentiated according to the Eight Principles, Yin and Yang, excess and deficiency, Qi and Blood, the theory of Zang-Fu organs, and the theory of meridians and collaterals. You will learn these concepts later."

They followed the Abbott through the temple toward Ma Guang Yah's room and Pei Ke's sudden silence told Liu that the boy was confused.

"Let me give you a good analogy of what I mean by a disruption of energy," he said. "Picture in your mind a large forest. Within that forest, streams of water bring nourishment to the plants and trees. Within our body, there are streams of energy bringing nourishment to all parts of our body. One day a large tree falls across one of these streams and blocks the flow. In our body, the streams of energy become blocked. If the water is blocked, the plants and trees downstream do not get enough water and will suffer. This is also true of the energy in our bodies. Just as there is a problem downstream, there is a problem upstream. The plants and trees are getting too much water, which can be just as bad. The same holds true for our bodies: when there is too much energy upstream, then there is a problem. The blockage can cause problems close to itself or anywhere along the pathway. It can even cause a problem along another pathway."

Pei Ke nodded, but he did not wait before asking another question.

"Then how do you as a doctor diagnose what is wrong?"

"Our ancestors were observant of cause and effect and what they observed has allowed us to make proper diagnoses. There were many good individuals like Huang Ti and Shen Nong, often referred to as the original founders of Chinese medicine. Huang Ti was part legend and part historical. He was, according to tradition, the founder of our people. Various historians claim he invented not only the calendar but also a system of telling time. He also composed the Yellow Emperor's Classic on Internal Medicine. This famous work is written in two parts. The first part is called Plain Questions. The second part is called the Spiritual Changeable Pivot. Both sections consist of a dialogue between Huang Ti and his minister, Chi Po. This book, though attributed to Huang Ti, is probably an accumulation of information passed down through the ages. I have seen a copy of this book.

"Shen Nung was famous for discovering various herbs. Another great contributor to Chinese medicine was Bian Que, who formulated the Four Basic Diagnostic Methods. From generation to generation, the accumulated knowledge was passed down in the form of verbal teachings and writings.

"Of course, many stories and legends exist to explain the origin of medicine itself. As with every legend, the exact facts may be lost or changed, but there is usually an underlying truth to the story. As it was passed on to me by my teachers, the beginning of how to heal came by accident. One day a small group of our ancestors gathered around a fire trying to keep warm when an ember from the fire flew and landed against the bottom of someone's foot. The heat from the ember stimulated an acupuncture point and that man's headache went away. Remember what I told you about the Yong Quan point on the bottom of the foot? Well, I suspect this point is where the ember landed. This point is used effectively in the treatment of headaches occurring on top of the head.

"Because our people settled in different regions of this country, medical knowledge evolved in diverse ways. Now we can categorize medical techniques by their origins. Acupuncture came from the Eastern area, while the treatment of internal problems with herbs originated in the Western part. The practice of exercise and breathing techniques like Tai Chi Chuan and Qi Gong came from the central region. Today an accomplished healer is well versed in acupuncture, herbs, Qi Gong, Tui Na, dietary considerations, and geomancy."

Pei Ke tried to look satisfied, but it was clear his question had not been answered.

"Master?"

"Yes?" Liu said.

"How do you actually make a diagnosis? I mean, what steps do you take?"

"There are both subjective and objective aspects of any diagnosis. The subjective aspect is what the patient relates to you, and the objective is what you find out from your examination. This is followed by the planned action you take, the prognosis, and the length of time it will take to get the desired results. In general, a diagnostic examination includes four elements: looking, listening and smelling, asking, and touching."

"Listening and smelling are in the same category?"

"Yes," Liu continued. "Now these four diagnostic tools are what Bian Que passed on to all of us so that we can treat patients. You are asking many questions. Do you want to become a martial artist or a doctor?"

Pei Ke thought for a few moments before replying. "Master, you are so well versed in martial arts, medicine, calligraphy, and painting. It would be nice to be able to do all those things. You must feel very proud of your knowledge and all your accomplishments."

"Pride only tricks your mind and sends the wrong message to those who know you. Yes, I do feel satisfaction, for each one of these arts follows within the tradition of being one with myself.

"Each of these arts lies within the person rather than lying outside of the person. They are a cultivation of knowledge and spirituality that leads to communion with the universal energy. Look at the animals. They appear peaceful within their own world. They follow what the universal Tao has set aside for them. Calm your mind and be peaceful with yourself and others. That is something you need to remember. A truly happy and peaceful person enjoys his own company and does not always need to be with others. It does not mean the person is a recluse or hermit, for interaction with other people is necessary for us to function within the Tao. Have you noticed those who always need the attention and company of others? They jump from one subject to another without pause. They seem to be everywhere. There is no true and lasting peacefulness to their minds."

Pei Ke nodded but his lips were pursed, as though he were resisting the urge to speak.

"Yes?" Liu said.

"Master, can we return to the subjective and objective aspects of diagnosis? How can just looking at someone help you arrive at a diagnosis?"

"Looking means to observe the external and unique characteristics of the patient, which convey the person's inner spirit and energy."

"What characteristics?"

"A patient's facial expression, how he walks, sits, stands, his manner of dress, the quality of his tongue, and the characteristics of his hair, eyes, skin, and nails. Even his stature will give you a clue as to the constitutional nature of the patient. For example, a person who is overweight tends to have a fat abdomen, and appears to walk slowly and easily becomes breathless. Master Ma is an example. He is overweight and he has breathing problems. For many overweight people, it is an indication of a phlegm problem with a basic spleen Qi deficiency. These are new terms for you and they have very specific meanings. I will discuss them with you when you are ready to understand diagnosis."

"Which one of the four diagnostic tools is the most important?"

"It is an accumulation of signs and symptoms that leads to a differential diagnosis and treatment plan. So, it is not just looking but rather looking, listening and smelling, asking, and touching. Looking is important, however. For example, looking at the patient's tongue can tell us what is happening inside the body."

"How?"

"The tongue has both a direct and an indirect connection with the internal organs of the body. It makes its connection through the meridian system. Changes taking place within the internal organs are reflected on the tongue. The tip of the tongue reflects what is happening with the heart. The center of the tongue reflects what is happening with the stomach and spleen. The left side of the tongue deals with the liver and the right side deals with the gallbladder. The back of the tongue deals with the kidney.

"Actually, you can also divide the tongue into three segments. The tip of the tongue deals with the upper part of the body, the middle of the tongue deals with the middle part of the abdomen, and the root or back of the tongue deals with the lower part of the abdomen. Think of the tongue as a book. Read the tongue for clues to help you further your diagnosis. The next time you have the chance you should look in a mirror and analyze your own tongue. The truly good doctor can make an accurate diagnosis by the observations I just mentioned."

"But what should I be looking for?"

"You should look at the color, shape, coating, and physical characteristics of the tongue. For example, a slightly pale tongue is normal. It is neither too pale nor too red. A tongue that is too pale is an indication of a coldness or deficiency in the body. A tongue that is overly red suggests an excess or heat condition in the body. A purple tongue indicates stagnation of blood.

"The shape of the tongue is also important. A swollen tongue is generally indicative of a spleen problem, usually with retention of some type of body fluids. A thin tongue can suggest a deficiency in the body or diminished fluids. Sometimes you will see a tongue with deep cracks along the surface. A cracked tongue can be normal if one is born with it. If one was not born with it then there is an internal problem

"In addition, the coating on the tongue is very important. It can be divided into two categories. The first is the quality of the coating. If it is thin, the disease process is at an early stage or on the outside or surface of the body. If it is thick, the disease has worked its way to the internal part of the body. A dry coating indicates heat or dehydration, while an excessively moist tongue indicates excessive mucus or dampness in the body.

"The second category is the color. A thin white coating is normal. However, it can also appear with cold or deficiency conditions. A yellow coating means that there are heat symptoms in the body—the deeper the yellow, and the thicker the coating, the more severe the disease process. A gray coating suggests deeper internal problems while a black coating indicates extreme conditions very often quite serious."

"There are so many things to remember," Pei Ke said.

Liu smiled.

"There are also markings on the tongue that can tell you what part of the body has a problem. For instance, if there are markings on the tip of the tongue or a very deep groove, there may be a heart issue. If the sides of the tongue appear to have teeth marks, it probably means a phlegm problem and that the patient may have other associated symptoms of mucus and bloatedness. I will explain more of this later. Just remember, always look at the tongue to help you with your diagnosis."

Pei Ke was silent for a moment and it was clear from his face that he was overwhelmed by all Liu had just said. It did not stop him from proceeding, however, and Liu nodded inwardly at the boy's desire to learn.

"Master," Pei Ke said with a deep breath. "You mentioned the diagnostic principle of listening. What are you listening for?"

"Actually I said that listening and smelling are combined as a means of diagnosis. You must listen more carefully."

"Yes Master," Pei Ke started to say, but Liu continued over him.

"As you know, the words listening and smelling are both written and pronounced the same. We differentiate the meaning by how they are used in context. That is one reason why we combine them into the same category.

"The way the patient breathes may indicate either excess or deficiency. A wheezing sound usually indicates a deficiency and a problem affecting the lung or kidney energy. The quality or sound of a cough is also very important. From the sound, you can differentiate a number of internal conditions.

"Odors from a body are important because they can indicate which meridian is unbalanced. For example, a goatish smell may indicate a gall bladder or liver energy problem; a fragrant smell, a spleen or stomach problem; a rancid smell, a lung or large intestine problem; a fishy rotten smell, a kidney or bladder problem; a burnt smell, a heart or small intestine problem."

"Master, you have covered two of the four. What is asking?"

"The patient's previous medical history, his current medical condition, his parents' medical history, and his lifestyle are all important things to know in the diagnostic process. To find out about these separate factors, the doctor should ask the patient a series of questions. The most important of these concern chills and fever, perspiration, urine and feces, diet and appetite, sleep, the condition of the chest and abdomen, the condition of the eyes and ears, and the overall health of the head and body.

"Often the answer to one question will lead you to another question, which in turn will trigger in the patient's mind an event or circumstance that helps you in your differential diagnosis."

He turned to Pei Ke.

"Again, I need to mention it is not just one of these factors that make a good diagnosis. Rather it is taking all these factors into consideration that makes for an exceptional doctor."

Pei Ke nodded.

"But Master," he said. "You've not said anything about the last principle, touching. How does it compare with the other three methods of diagnosis?"

"Good," Liu said, complimenting the boy's memory. "Touching has three components. The first is to palpate the body to feel if there are any hard masses, swelling, hot or cold areas, depressions, pain or tenderness, and so on. Usually, but not always, the patient indicates that a certain area of his body has a problem, which would lead you to feel that area. For example, the patient may tell you his right knee hurts. When you touch his right knee, if it is warmer than the left, you might suspect that there is an excess condition. Why?"

"Because heat suggests an excess?"

"Good. The second component of touching involves applying pressure to areas of the body for diagnostic purposes. For example, acupuncture points along the Urinary Bladder Meridian, which runs bilateral to the spine, can be used for diagnosis and treatment. These points are referred to as Shu Points. As an example, the acupuncture point Fei Shu can be used as a diagnostic point as well as a treatment point for lung problems. As a diagnostic point, it will be tender to the touch.

"This is the situation with Master Ma and his asthma. As a treatment point, the doctor can insert a needle into this point to help relieve the asthmatic symptoms. Each of these Shu Points is associated with an internal organ, and each organ is associated with a specific meridian. If the points are tender to the touch, it may indicate an imbalance of energy in that specific organ or meridian. Another example of a Shu Point is Wei Shu. If it is tender or sore to the touch, it may denote gastric problems. Using acupuncture on this point may relieve the gastric symptoms.

"In addition, when these Shu Points are painful to the touch, it may indicate problems in the sensory organs, which are related to the internal organs. For example, the eyes are governed by the liver, and it would be appropriate to use the acupuncture point Gan Shu for treating eye diseases.

"We refer to some acupuncture points as Mu points. They are located on the chest and abdomen, and are associated with specific internal organs. Their tenderness upon palpation is indicative of internal problems. As an example, the acupuncture point Zhong Wan is located above the umbilicus. It is very effective for treating chronic stomach or gastric problems.

"Basically, the Mu points relate to Yin and the Shu points relate to Yang. However, to treat a disease of the Yin organs we could choose points on the back and to treat diseases of the Yang organs we could choose points on the abdomen and chest. This is an example of choosing Yin to treat Yang and Yang to treat Yin.

"In addition to the Mu and Shu points, points exist along the side of the fingernails and toenails, next to the cuticle. These are referred to as the Bubbling Well points and they are the beginning or end of the flow of energy along a meridian. These points can also be used for diagnosis and treatment. Tenderness at these points indicates an imbalance of energy pertaining to that particular meridian. Squeezing these points may assist in finding which meridian is out of balance."

"Master, how do you squeeze these points?"

"It is done the same for all the fingers and toes. Use the thumb and the index finger, hold, and squeeze both sides of the finger close to the cuticle. Always apply the same amount of pressure on each finger or toe. Ask the patient if it hurts, and which one hurts the most. Usually the patient will be able to tell you that one finger hurts more than another."

"And the finger that hurts the most has the greatest imbalance?"

"Correct, though it does not necessarily mean that there is a problem with the organ itself. If the index finger is the most reactive it could mean there is a large intestine related problem. It could also mean the energy of the Large Intestine Meridian is out of balance, affecting another meridian and or the internal organ. Do you understand the difference?"

"Yes, Master. But which fingers are associated with which meridians?"

"When you learn the pathway of the flow of energy, you will learn which finger and toe is associated with which meridian. Basically, all the energy of the Yin meridians on the arm flow from the chest to the fingers and all the energy of the Yang meridians on the arm flow from the fingers to the chest. The energy of the Yin meridians on the legs flow from the toes to the trunk and the energy of the Yang meridians on the legs flow from the head to the toes."

"Master, how am I going to remember all this?"

"It requires a lot of memorization on your part. And you will need to pay attention."

"Yes, Master."

"In addition to the Well points, there are Ashi points, which become sore if there is a problem with the flow of energy. Don't confuse this soreness with normal bruises.

"Ashi points were first discussed by Sun Si Mao. He lived in the Tang Dynasty. He believed there was energy throughout the body and whenever there was any type of soreness or discomfort, there was an acupuncture point. These points did not necessarily have to be on the meridian system; they could be anywhere on the body. When locating points, it helps to know the nature of the soreness, and whether or not it is a regular acupuncture point or an Ashi Point. In general, if the soreness of the point is dull when palpated, it is possibly a Yin problem. If the pain on palpation is very sharp, then it is most likely a Yang problem."

"Master, sometimes I have pain in my abdomen. Would that be an Ashi point?"

"Is the pain on the surface and muscles or is it deep inside the abdomen?"

"It is deep inside the abdomen."

"In that case, it is probably not an Ashi Point. Basically, if there is pain on palpation, there is an imbalance of energy and it needs to be investigated further through other diagnostic procedures. If there is a mass on palpating the abdomen, it could be either a blockage of Qi or Blood."

Pei Ke began pushing his fingers into his belly experimentally.

"Master, when palpating the abdomen, how much pressure should be applied?"

"If the patient already knows there is pain in the abdomen, it is not wise to immediately apply force."

Pei Ke pulled his hand away quickly.

Liu continued: "It is better to start gently and to question the patient on the amount of pain. If the patient does not initially tell you there is pain, then you can press on different areas of the abdomen and gently apply pressure. A good rule for you to follow is to go slowly and gently until you understand what you are doing or until you understand what the patient is telling you. Do you understand?"

"Yes, Master."

"Good. Then I will move on. The third type of touching is referred to as pulse diagnosis. The concept of using the radial artery for pulse diagnosis was discovered by Wang Shu-Ho. The pulses are felt along the radial artery at the wrist. There are different schools of thought on how the pulses are taken, but this is neither the time nor the place to get into that.

"Basically, there are three sites on each wrist to feel at three different depths with twenty-eight separate qualities. To feel the pulses, you need to first put your middle finger on the styloid process on the radial side of the wrist."

Pei Ke moved a hand to his wrist, hesitated, then looked at his master.

"The styloid process is the bony protrusion on the inside of your wrist," Liu said patiently, "about one half inch above your wrist crease on the same side as your thumb. I want you to do that as we are walking.

"With the palm of your left hand facing toward you, place the palm of your right hand around the outside of your left wrist. Curl your fingers over the side of the wrist to the radial artery. Do you feel your pulses?"

"Yes, Master. I can feel the throbbing of the pulse. It feels like the beating of a drum."

"Good, remember to always place the pad of the middle finger first on the protruding bone, followed by placing the pad of the index finger next to it and then the same with the ring finger on the other side. The first contact point you make with the middle finger is called the Guan point, followed by the Cun point, and the Chi point. I want you to do this now, so that I can watch."

"Master, am I supposed to feel them all at one time or separately?"

"You need to first feel the Guan Point. Once you can feel that energy flowing, then release the pressure on the artery and then feel the Cun Point followed by the Chi Point. Try that now and tell me what you feel."

Liu watched as his student slowly arranged his fingers as instructed. He was certainly willing to do what he was asked.

"Master, they feel different."

"Yes. Tell me how."

"I do not know how to explain it adequately, but one of them feels very strong and the other two do not feel quite as strong, almost as if there is softness to the drum beat. Is there something wrong with me?"

"No, there is nothing wrong with you in the context of what you are thinking. Many people have an imbalance of energy at any one point in time.

"Now with your middle finger back on the Guan Point, I want you to apply a little pressure to the point. Do you feel a difference in the pulse between just resting your finger on the point, then putting more pressure on the point?"

"Yes, Master, there is a distinct difference between them."

"What is that difference?"

"When I just rested my finger on the pulse, the beat is not as firm or strong as when I apply a little more pressure. There is actually a distinct difference between the two beats."

"There are actually three levels to the pulse. The first is the superficial level and can be felt by simply resting your finger on the artery. The second, middle level can be felt by applying a little more pressure, and the third level, what we call the deep level, can be felt when you apply even greater pressure.

"The superficial level corresponds to the condition of the Yang organs. The middle level corresponds to the condition or state of Blood. The deep level corresponds to the condition of the Yin organs. It is my opinion that the superficial level pertains to the Heavens, the middle level pertains to Man, and the deep level pertains to the Earth, though others might disagree."

He ignored his student's expression of awe.

"Pulse diagnosis is a very difficult technique to master," Liu said. "Often a doctor spends years of practice in feeling the pulses to become expert with this technique. For your initial training, you need only to distinguish between the superficial and deep pulses. As you gain more experience, you can divide the pulses into the three depths."

"Master, it seems you mentioned qualities as well."

"Yes," Liu said. "There are twenty-eight qualities of these pulses that you need to remember: superficial, deep, slow, rapid, deficient, excess, surging, thready, rolling, hesitant, string-taut, tense, soft, weak, abrupt, knotted, hollow, scattered, moving, stiff, concealed, wiry, overflowing, short, long, full, empty, and slippery.

"In addition, these twenty-eight qualities can be grouped into categories such as floating, deep, slow, rapid, empty, and full. These six categories can be further classified as either excess or deficient. Ultimately you are feeling the pulses to determine if there is an excess or deficiency in the patient's body. The beginning student must be able to differentiate these two conditions. Once you are able to distinguish between excess and deficiency, then understanding the six categories will help you to further differentiate the full extent of either the Yin or the Yang. Isolating exactly each of the twenty-eight pulses will help you differentiate the extent of the problem. Learning how to do this takes time."

"Master, will you show me how to correctly differentiate the pulses?"

"Of course, but for now just listen. Everything at its appropriate time."

"Yes, Master."

"Each pulse corresponds to a specific organ of the body. On the right-hand side, the superficial Cun pulse corresponds to the large intestine while the deep pulse corresponds to the lung. The superficial Guan pulse corresponds to the stomach while the deep pulse corresponds to the spleen. On the Chi pulse, the superficial level pertains to the urinary bladder and the deeper pulse pertains to the kidney.

"On the left-hand side, the Cun pulse at the superficial level pertains to the small intestine and the deep level to the heart. At the Guan position, the superficial pulse pertains to the gall bladder and the deep pulse to the liver. On the Chi pulse, the superficial level pertains to the triple warmer and the deep level to the kidney. Basically, the Cun, Guan, and Chi pulses refer to the upper, middle, and lower portions of the trunk of the body. Remember these pulses refer to both the organs of the body and the energy of the meridians associated with the particular organ.

"To help you remember which pulse belongs to which organ, think of Yin and Yang. The superficial pulses are associated with the Yang organs. The deep pulses are associated with the Yin organs."

"Master, how long did it take for you to become proficient in this technique?"

"Since this technique is one of the most difficult of all the diagnostic techniques, it takes the longest time to master. I don't think anyone ever fully masters the technique. They only get better over time. This is the joy in doing this diagnostic technique. It is always a challenge to discover the correct reading in diagnosing the condition of the patient.

"If your reading of the pulse is wrong, there is a good chance your diagnosis will be wrong. Therefore, your treatment protocol will be wrong and the patient will not benefit from the treatment. A wrong treatment protocol could, in some situations, aggravate the condition.

"Many times doctors ask themselves why the patient did not get well. The answer in many instances is not that the patient did not respond to the treatment protocol, but rather that the diagnosis was wrong from the beginning.

"The reading of the pulses indicates what is occurring within internal organs, and whether there is an excess or deficiency of energy. It is important that the patient is relaxed when you take his pulse. You should not hurry the pulse diagnosis or you may arrive at the wrong conclusion. The patient should be sitting if possible, or lying down, and should be resting for a few minutes before you take his pulse. His wrist should be at the same level as the heart. Never take a pulse without the patient first resting, as you will almost always get an exaggerated indication due to the patient's accelerated heart rate."

"Master, do all doctors take the pulses in the same way as you?"

"No, there are different schools of thought on pulse diagnosis. Once you become somewhat proficient with this method, you can learn other philosophies on taking the pulses. Sometimes it is necessary to switch from one method to another; however, remember that, essentially, all pulse taking is the same. In ancient times there were other locations on the body used to take the pulses, but those techniques are either lost or have gone out of favor."

"Master...."

"Enough for the moment. Let's hurry to see Ma Guang Yah."

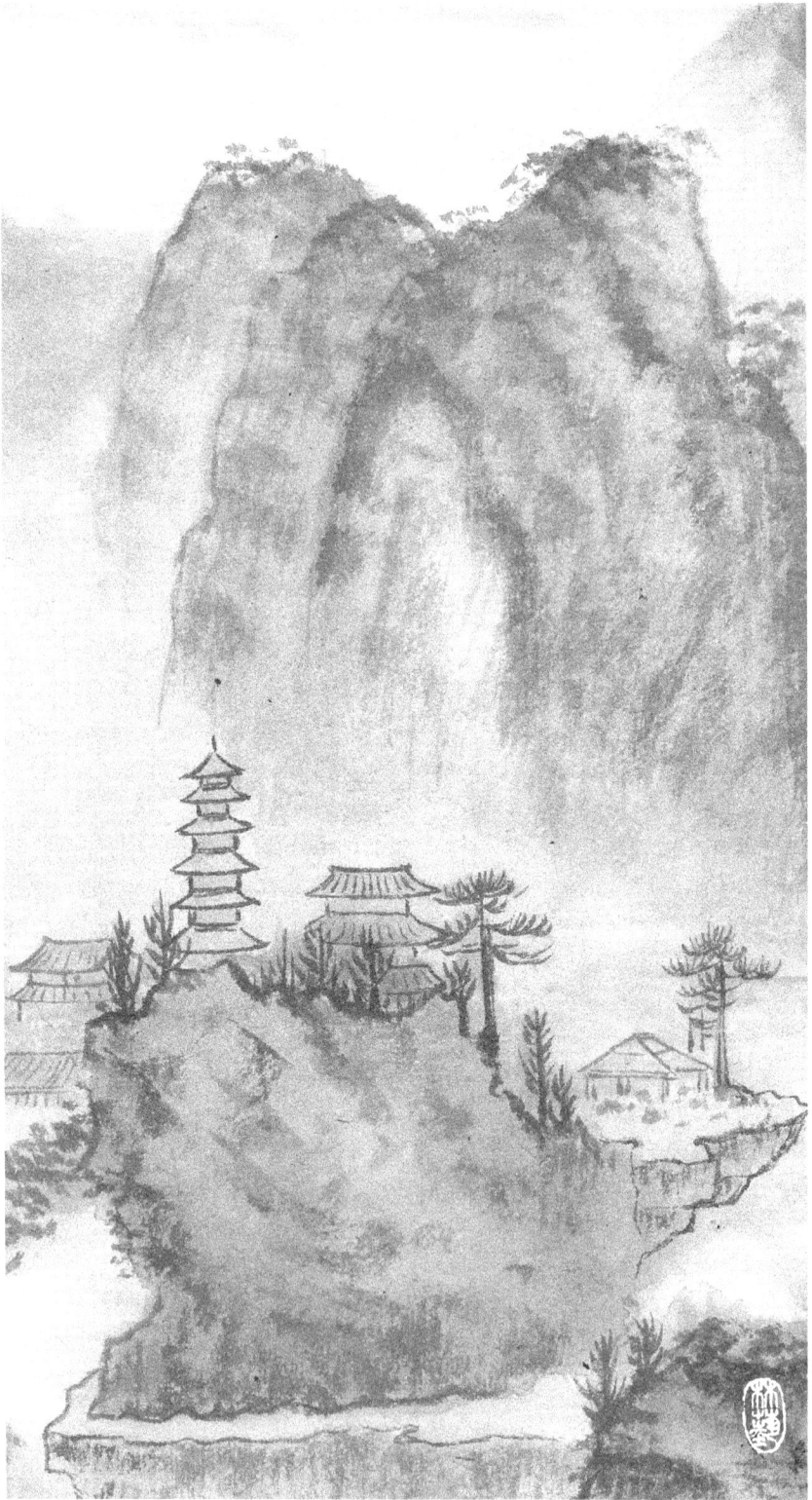

# CHAPTER THREE

"Pei Ke."

"Yes, Master."

The two men, Liu and Pei Ke, were finishing their mid-day meal and were preparing to leave the temple.

"Do you have the sack and all the things I gave you to carry?"

"Yes, Master. I put everything in the sack as you requested."

"And all the little things I gave you to carry? Are they with you also?"

"Yes, Master. I have taken care to make sure everything is safe and accounted for. I've not forgotten anything, nor left anything behind."

"Good. You must safeguard the sack and its contents at all times. I want you to wear this amulet around your neck."

"What is it for," asked Pei Ke as he looked at the amulet.

"It is for good luck. If for some reason we get separated on our journey, just take the amulet to the Abbot in my ancestral village. He will know who gave it to you."

"Master, it looks like it is broken."

"Yes, I know."

Pei Ke put the amulet around his neck. He realized he had just agreed to carry both his master's things and his own. He was not sure why it bothered him. Master Liu is my teacher. He is testing to see if I am dedicated.

Pei Ke wondered why they were suddenly going on this journey. What had the letter said? Why had Liu been summoned to the valley of his nativity? He also wondered about Liu's family. What would they think of him? He realized that he was hoping to find a place of belonging at the end of their journey. He had never been more than a day from his birthplace and thoughts of the world beyond that border made him both excited and nervous.

"Master," he said timidly. "Where is your ancestral village? How long will we be traveling before we get there?"

Liu smiled faintly and Pei Ke thought the master's hand drifted briefly to the pocket where Liu kept the message he had received the day before.

"It will take us nearly a fortnight," he answered. "We will travel as quickly as we can, but there are places we will need to stop. If we are lucky, someone with a cart will give us a ride."

His hand drifted to the message again and Pei Ke wondered once more what it said.

"My family, going back many generations, lives in Hebei Province," Liu continued. "Actually, I am the first to leave and live so far away. The land there is very mountainous, but my brother lives in a valley. Our route is the same as that of generations of travelers and we will meet many different people."

He looked in the direction of his home. Pei Ke suspected that his master had not visited his home in many years and he wondered what they would find there.

"I do not think we will meet with any problems," Liu said suddenly, turning to face his student. "But it is not an easy journey. It is still early autumn and so there should not be any snow or sleet, but even so, many who have traveled this route have died due to the weather." He paused, then said, "Are you sure you want to accompany me? It may be dangerous for you, and you will be a long way from home and friends. You may stay behind and wait for me to return, if you wish."

Pei Ke thought for a minute. Master Liu possessed nothing but the clothes on his back and the things in his pack. There was no reason for him to return. Pei Ke felt suddenly that the world of his future had been put in a bowl and was being handed to him. He took a deep breath, looked his master in the eyes, and answered.

"My parents died a long time ago," he said, "and there was nothing for me to inherit, not after the disease that took them. The money went to the doctors. My older sister is married and lives with her husband and mother-in-law. My brother died while I was very young. Any friends I leave will always be friends. There is nothing really to keep me here, but much to gain if I join you. Where you go, I will go." Pei Ke looked at Liu, waiting for a favorable response.

"Why are you so intent on learning martial arts? There are many other things you could do that would be just as honorable."

"You have asked me that question before, Master."

"Yes, and I ask you again. Why do you want to learn martial arts?"

"I've been fascinated with it since I saw a group of dancers come through the village." Pei Ke smiled ruefully. "I wanted to join then, but they laughed and said I was too skinny."

Liu looked at Pei Ke and mentally agreed. He had thought many times before that the boy's stature would need some improving if he really wanted to be good in martial arts. It was not the bulk but the fitness that was necessary to do well in the internal martial arts.

"A real scholar learns more than martial arts," Liu said out loud. "He also learns medicine, calligraphy, painting, and the classic works of Lao Tzu, Confucius, and Buddha."

Liu looked at Pei Ke intently.

"If you choose to come with me, things will be different. You will no longer be just a student, but my disciple. There will be many hardships for you to endure—many more than you have experienced so far. There will be times you will want to quit but will have to forge onward. There will be times you will be asked to do things that may or may not have an apparent reason. I expect you to do them without question. There will be times when you will question everything told you. You will not believe some of the things you are taught, but you must accept them. There will be times when the training will seem almost unbearable, but you must know that I will not ask you to do anything that I have not done in the past nor anything that I am not capable of doing now. You will be following ancient travels of the mind, body, and soul. Is this what you want? It will require complete loyalty." There was a question to this final statement.

"I agree," said Pei Ke immediately. He bowed low in respect. He felt a chill go through his body as he realized that he had just embarked on a new life.

Liu wondered if Pei Ke's eagerness was a sign of his respect for what lay ahead or if it only marked a desire to learn how to fight. Did he really understand what lay ahead? Did he have the internal fortitude and stamina to handle the training he would undergo? These and other questions went through Liu's mind as he gave his good-byes to those in the temple. He sensed this farewell would last a long time.

As he and Pei Ke started toward the distant mountains and his home, Liu thought again of the letter in his pocket. The messenger had demanded no fee, so either he had been paid in advance or he was to be paid at the conclusion of the delivery. Someone was waiting for something to happen, but who and what?

No seal marked the note. Its writing appeared hurried, as if the writer had been agitated. From the way it was written, Liu could tell the composer of the message was somewhat educated. He did not recognize the name at the bottom of the note, but he knew whoever had written it had personal knowledge of the Liu family. The note mentioned his brother, members of the family, and servants and the author claimed that he held these captive. The note requested a ransom to guarantee their safe release, though it would be impossible to hold everyone for ransom and expect Liu to have the money to pay them. Why had the messenger been so nervous? His brother hadn't written the note, though if his brother were being held for ransom, it seemed as though it would be logical to force him to write the note. Something was wrong with his family.

Looking at his new disciple, he tried to put thoughts of his brother from his head. Pei Ke shifted the weight on his back to make it more comfortable. Neither of them looked back at the temple.

"Pei Ke," Liu said. "We learn martial arts to train the mind, body, and spirit, we train our minds to be disciplined, our bodies to provide us with a long healthy life, and our spirit to make us one with the universe. Cherish all forms of life, for all living things have a place and purpose on this earth. We must blend into the overall scheme of an ever-changing universe. We hold all life to be sacred, even the life of the lowliest creatures. We do not eat meat nor do we take any animal's life."

"Master, if someone attacks me, what do I do to protect myself?"

"You have the right and obligation to protect yourself at all times, but the force you use must be just enough so the attacker is not permanently hurt. Don't let your anger or emotions get in the way when you are confronted with an adversary."

"What do I do and how do I do it? What if he wants to kill me?"

"The answer will be there when you need to know. Remember to hold all life sacred."

Pei Ke thought it was an impossible situation. He was to protect himself but not to hurt anyone. He wondered if the master had ever had to defend himself. He had heard that Master Liu was a proficient in the things he knew, but stories were often enhanced with each telling. Pei Ke remembered the Abbot saying that once a group of thieves came to the temple to steal some statues. The master had been asleep at the time, but was aroused by the commotion. Each monk told a different story, but Pei Ke assumed the thieves fled after Master Liu had shown them a few examples of his skill. Pei Ke wished he had been there to see it.

The road to Liu's ancestral village led the two travelers north to the nearest village. This main road provided a means for the outlying farmers to take their produce to market. As the road sloped downward, the vegetation changed from bamboo forest to productive farmland.

Each farmer had his own piece of land, usually separated from his neighbor's by a long tree line or a stand of bamboo. Farmers grew rice in the fields, which was their main staple. Each house had a large garden that supplied the necessary vegetables. Nearby pens housed the cows, pigs, ducks, and chickens. This scene repeated itself continually as they walked together towards the village.

"Master," Pei Ke said softly as he turned around to look. "I think someone is following us."

"Actually, two people have been following us since we left the temple."

"How did you know that?"

"Some of the villagers told the Abbot who in turn told me before we left that there were two strangers asking about the temple and me. We don't often have strangers in this area. They usually make the villagers uneasy. I noticed them following us shortly after we left."

"Why are they following us?"

"I do not know."

"Should we be concerned?" Again Pei Ke turned to look behind. He wished that he knew who the strangers were and why they were following them.

"I don't think they will bother us."

Pei Ke turned his attention to the fields, trying to put thoughts of strange men following them from his head. Finally he turned to the master.

"Master, we have some time before we get to the village. May I ask you some questions concerning medicine?"

Times have really changed, Liu thought. When he had studied, he would never have thought to ask his teacher any questions. It would have been extremely impolite and any teacher would have punished him. On the other hand, he had been eager to learn just as Pei Ke was. Liu wondered if he should hold the boy back or encourage him to ask.

"You may ask me one question."

"When Master Ma was sick and could not breathe, how did you know what was wrong?"

Liu chuckled to himself. The boy had asked a single question, but the answer could go on for several days.

"There is not a simple answer to your question. Do you remember when you asked me about how to diagnose and I told you the basic principles?"

"Yes Master."

"Well, tell me."

"The first thing we need to do is to observe the patient."

"That is correct. What did you observe when we were with Master Ma?"

"He was lying down."

"Why was he lying down?"

"Master, he looked weak, which could explain it."

"Good. What else did you observe?"

"It was difficult for him to breathe."

"Correct. What else?"

"I observed nothing else, Master."

"You did not observe that the color of his skin was slightly chalky and that he had a sense of apprehension in his voice? From observing him in the past, I noticed that he did not usually walk very fast. His tongue seemed pale, which indicates there is an underlying deficiency. I will explain all this to you later. Now, Pei Ke, what did you hear?"

Liu looked at Pei Ke, and Pei Ke was uncertain about what to say.

"Nothing, Master."

"If you listened carefully you would have heard a wheezing sound coming from Ma. The wheezing indicated that it is difficult for him to exhale. What did you smell?"

"Nothing Master."

"Pei Ke, do you remember what I asked Ma?"

"Yes, Master. You asked him if there was any pain or discomfort in his chest, abdomen, or legs."

"Do you remember that I felt his chest, legs, and abdomen?"

"Yes, Master."

"When I felt his chest I was trying to find out if the acupuncture points from the center of his chest to his throat were sore to my touch. In most asthma patients, these points are sore and you can tonify these points with acupressure or acupuncture. This temporarily relieves the asthmatic symptoms. The acupuncture points along the medial aspect of his calf were also sore. The inside of the leg is where the spleen, kidney, and liver meridians are located. They are Yin meridians, and flow from the foot upward to the body. In many instances, if points in this area are sore then the inside of the leg can be a good diagnostic tool. Many of these points will also be Ashi Points. As I told you before an Ashi Point is a spontaneous sore point not usually on the meridian system. Points that are sore can indicate a deficiency. You can tonify these points by inserting the needle in the direction of the energy flow. The ancient textbooks indicate that asthma can be due to a kidney problem and not necessarily a lung problem. The pulse diagnosis will be one of the major factors in the diagnosis of what ails Mr. Ma.

"As you insert each needle into the Ashi Point, ask the patient if his lungs feel better. Often the patient will be able to indicate a certain area of the chest that now seems more open. Once you understand the relationship between the area on the medial aspect of the lower leg and the area of the chest to which it corresponds, then you can direct your needling to concentrate on that area where the chest constriction is the worst.

"This also works for back pain. When someone has pain anywhere from their tail bone to their neck, but cannot lie on their abdomen, you can treat the back pain by having them lie on their back and put needles along the medial aspect of the calf. The area near the anklebone corresponds with the tailbone and the area below the knee corresponds with the neck. Begin the procedure by inserting a needle in San Yin Jiao followed by a needle in the first Ashi Point near the ankle bone. Insert the needles in the direction of the energy flow. As you put needles into each succeeding Ashi Point, the patient will feel a warming sensation. This starts in his leg, then moves to the tailbone, and finally rises up the spine and back. The patient will have an overall feeling of deep relaxation. When you ask him if it feels like melting butter, he will agree. His hips will open up and relax. The tension in the neck and shoulders will disappear."

"Master?"

"Yes."

"I'm confused. If I understand you correctly; when someone has a kidney problem, he always has pain along the inside of the lower leg, and it causes asthma and back pain."

"You are partially correct. First, if someone has kidney problems, he may not have any lung problems or back pain. Some people will have either asthma or back pain or both, but not all people. Now I will ask your next question for you: who will have asthma, who will have back pain, and who will have both? The answer lies in a number of complicated factors. One of the most important factors is that person's constitution at birth. If an individual is predisposed to having one or more health-related issues, then there will be a problem associated with the energy of the meridian involved. That person then stands a good chance of having some problems. For example, if you were born with a tendency for issues in the lower back and if you then develop a kidney deficiency, you will probably have back pain."

"How do you know if or when you will have a problem?" Pei Ke felt his lower back and wondered if he had a problem. He remembered his father would always complain of low back pain.

"You will never know for sure, but there is a way to get some idea of your excesses and deficiencies."

"You mean you can tell me right now where and when I am going to have a health concern."

"Not exactly. Based on your date and time of birth, the heavens and earth had an influence on you the moment you were born. Most people have a combination of excesses and deficiencies at birth. Some scholars can tell you this by looking up your birthday. There is a special book that lists birthdates."

"Master, this is why I want to study and learn from you. This is fascinating. Can you predict these influences?"

"I can tell you general tendencies. It is up to you to lead a lifestyle that will be conducive to your health. However, I do not have a copy of the book I need with me. It is at the temple for the monks. Part of your training will be to learn to diagnose using this constitutional theory. You will learn that theory later. It is all part of the theory of Yin and Yang."

"Master, I remember my school teachers and parents telling me about the concepts of Yin and Yang."

"You should have paid more attention when you were young. The concepts of Yin and Yang are Taoist. They pertain to everything in our culture and date back as far as the Book of Changes written during the Zhou Dynasty. Their foundation comes from Lao Tzu, the great philosopher, who wrote the Tao Te Ching. They permeate all facets of medicine. Yin and Yang have come to be known as complimentary opposites. Each one exists because the other exists. For example, there is a positive and a negative. You would not know what positive was unless you knew what negative was. In addition, there is the concept of up. You would not know what up was unless you had some knowledge of down. Do you understand?"

"Yes, Master. It is like left and right, North and South, East and West, male and female."

"Correct. However, it is much more than that. Even though they are opposites, taken together they form a whole entity. Within itself, the two parts are complimentary and dependent. Within Yin there is a little bit of Yang and within Yang there is a little bit of Yin. There is nothing categorized as being totally Yin or Yang. To complicate the matter, when Yin goes to the extreme, it becomes Yang and when Yang goes to the extreme it becomes Yin. In addition, they mutually consume each other or replace the other. If Yin increases then Yang decreases and if Yin decreases then Yang increases. You will often see this in the progression of a disease. The disease will progress from a Yin stage to a Yang stage."

"Master, can you give me an example?"

"Yes, when you have the first signs of fever you may be cold, but it is later followed by heat. Knowing the stage of the disease can help you treat the problem. You would not give cooling herbs if the patient had cold symptoms and you would not give warming herbs if the patient had hot symptoms. In medicine, we are concerned with specific examples of these complementary opposites. We are especially concerned with interior versus exterior, hot versus cold, rising versus sinking, damp versus dry, and expanding versus contracting, as well as tonification and depletion, weak and strong, hard and soft, fast and slow, and substantial and insubstantial."

"Master, how many acupuncture points are there on the body?"

Liu sighed. The boy's head jumped around with exasperating speed.

"Pei Ke, your mind is not focused. You are moving from one subject to another. Try to focus on the subject at hand at the moment."

"I'm sorry, Master. I have so many questions I want to ask, and I can't ask them all at the same time."

"To answer your question, there are many acupuncture points on the body, and there are new ones being discovered each year. The basic primary meridian system, which all acupuncturists memorize, has a fixed number of three hundred sixty-one acupuncture points. Legend, however, suggests there are three hundred sixty-five acupuncture points on the basic meridian system—one point for each day of the year. It is generally thought that the location of four points have been lost, though I think I know where at least one of them is and maybe two more.

"It can become very confusing to understand all the points so it is best to first understand the meridian system and leave the acupuncture points for later. For example, there are Twelve Main Meridians on the body. These are bilateral, which means they are on both the left and right sides of the body. There are also two singular meridians. One of the singular meridians is located on the front centerline of the body and the other is on the back centerline of the body. Each meridian has a connection to another meridian so there is a constant flow of energy throughout the body. Together the

Twelve Main Meridians and two single meridians are called the System of Fourteen Meridians. You will need to memorize these meridians. To make things more confusing, other meridian systems exist in the body, but your primary concern is to memorize the fourteen meridians. Later you can memorize the other meridian systems."

"If there is a constant flow of energy, where does the energy start?" Pei Ke said, swatting at an insect that seemed to take a liking to his face. Then he remembered what the master had said about valuing life and he put his hands behind his back.

"No real starting point exists on the body," Master Liu said, "but for generations doctors have used a model to better understand this flow. Think of the energy as being circular. It flows continuously around the circuit every twenty-four hours."

"So the energy never starts and stops?"

"Don't interrupt, just listen."

"Sorry, Master."

"The question of where the energy starts has come up before. To help us better understand the flow we will assume the most critical aspect of our life is the air we breathe. We will use the lungs as our starting point. Energy associated with the lungs is called lung energy. This lung energy flows on a meridian in our body called the Lung Meridian. The lung energy flows into the Large Intestine Meridian. The sequence continues in this order: lung, large intestine, stomach, spleen, heart, small intestine, bladder, kidney, pericardium, triple warmer, gall bladder, and liver. When the energy arrives at the end of the Liver Meridian, twenty-four hours have elapsed. This energy then flows into the starting point of the Lung Meridian to start the circular flow once again. Think of the energy flow as water going around a circular tube. There is no beginning nor is there an end to the energy. It is just there in a continuous cycle.

"Half of these meridians are Yin and half are Yang. The Yin meridians are lung, spleen, heart, kidney, pericardium, and liver. The Yang meridians are large intestine, stomach, small intestine, bladder, triple warmer, and gall bladder.

"Each Yin meridian connects to a Yang meridian in this circular flow. Thus, lung which is Yin is connected to large intestine which is Yang. This gives us a complimentary pair of Yin and Yang. The last Yang meridian is gall bladder and it connects to liver, which is its Yin partner. The energy then starts over again as I mentioned before and goes from liver to lung to start another twenty-four hour cycle."

"Master, you mentioned Pericardium Meridian and Triple Warmer Meridian. I have never heard of these organs."

"The pericardium surrounds your heart. The triple warmer is not an organ in the body but rather a segmentation of the trunk of the body into three separate areas. There are the upper, middle, and lower warmers."

Pei Ke looked confused and though Liu sensed the confusion, he did not provide an explanation, so Pei Ke asked another question.

"Master, you mentioned the end of the Liver Meridian. There must be a beginning and an end to each meridian."

"Yes, there is a beginning and an end to each meridian."

"How does the energy of one meridian get to the beginning of another meridian?"

"A segment of energy flow connects one meridian to another. This connection, however, is not necessarily at the end of the meridian. For example, the first acupuncture point for the Lung Meridian starts at a depression on the front of the chest just below the collarbone and close to the shoulder. It flows down the inside of the arm to the last acupuncture point at the cuticle on the side of the thumb. The first acupuncture point of the Large Intestine Meridian, which is the next meridian, is at the cuticle on the side of the index finger. The energy cannot jump from the cuticle of the thumb to the cuticle of the index finger. An acupuncture point just above the wrist on the Lung Meridian called Lie Que is where the energy connects from the Lung Meridian to the Large Intestine Meridian. This energy pathway is an internal pathway. The energy travels from Lie Que across the hand directly to the first acupuncture point of the Large Intestine Meridian."

"Master, I am confused. The energy of the Lung Meridian goes from the collar bone area to the thumb. If I understand you correctly, it also connects to a point of energy just above the wrist and travels to the Large Intestine Meridian on the index finger. How does the energy get to the thumb? Isn't it diverted to the index finger?"

"Remember my example of how energy is like water in a circular tube." Liu moved his arms in a big circle.

"Yes."

"Think of the energy in the Lung Meridian as being water. The water flows down the arm to Lie Que acupuncture point and continues to the thumb. However, the water also branches out from Lie Que and goes to the first point of the Large Intestine Meridian. The energy is in both places. Every meridian connects to another meridian. You can think of the pathway of the Lung Meridian as external and the connection between meridians as being internal. No acupuncture points exist between the connections.

"In addition, internal pathways connect the meridian to its specific organ. As an example, remember I told you that the first acupuncture point on the Lung Meridian starts just below the collarbone next to the front of the shoulder?"

"Yes, Master."

"There is an internal pathway for the Lung Meridian that has no acupuncture points. This pathway starts in the middle of the abdomen and descends along the center of the body to the large intestine. Remember the large intestine follows the lung in the circular flow of energy?"

"Yes, Master."

"After energy intersects with the large intestine, it then rises upwards, separates, and enters into each lung energizing the lungs. Then the energy returns to the centerline, rises upwards to the throat and separates into two pathways. One goes to the first acupuncture point of the Lung Meridian on the right side and the other goes to the first acupuncture point of the Lung Meridian on the left side. Remember that the twelve meridians are bilateral, meaning that they exist on both sides."

"Yes, Master. I remember. But what is this energy that you keep speaking of?"

"The energy or Qi is the life force keeping you and me alive. At the moment when this life force becomes totally used up, depleted, or exhausted, we die. However, ways exist to ensure this energy does not become fully consumed. In other words, we get our Qi from eating the right foods and herbs, drinking the right liquids, getting the appropriate rest, practicing moderation in sexual activities, and doing Tai Chi Chuan and or Qi Gong."

"Master, is that why you do Tai Chi Chuan and the basic Qi Gong exercises?" As he asked the question he already knew the answer.

"Yes. Tai Chi Chuan and the basic Qi Gong exercises are fundamental for a long healthy life."

"Master...."

"Pei Ke, you have too many questions. Just listen. Only one type of Qi exists, but it manifests itself in many different ways. They are easy to confuse, especially since they are used in different concepts. When we talk about medicine, we talk about one concept of Qi. When we talk about martial arts, we discuss another concept of Qi. As an example, we have discussed the flow of energy in the Lung Meridian. Well, this flow is Qi.

"The first Qi you acquired is called Primordial Qi. It is the energy instilled in you at conception. This is the Qi that determined who you became. It came from both of your parents. It included Qi from your grandparents, great grandparents, and so on. You have heard that children sometimes look and act like their parents or grandparents. This similarity is one small aspect of the Qi parents pass on to their children. This Qi stays with a child the rest of his life. He in turn will pass some of the Qi onto his sons and daughters when he has a family.

"The second type of Qi is Post Heaven Qi. This is the Qi originating from the liquids we drink and the food we eat. The Qi is produced by the stomach and spleen. That is why we need to eat the right foods and to do so in moderation. As an example, eating only one type of food will not properly allow the Post Heaven Qi to develop. Food that is tainted in any way will also hamper the development of this Post Heaven Qi. Our development physically, mentally, and spiritually will depend on what we put into our bodies. Do not smoke opium or take drugs and do not drink any fermented beverages. You should remember, Pei Ke, to treat your body as if it is a Taoist temple. You would never deface the temple; so don't defile your body.

"The third type of Qi is a combination of the Qi coming from our parents and the Qi we get from the air we breathe and from the food and liquids we take into our body. It is believed the Qi is stored in our kidneys, the area between our kidneys, and circulates throughout our body. It is the underlying basis for our development from the time we were born until the time we die. In actuality, the depletion of this energy is considered by many scholars to be the one of the reasons we die. The development of this Qi is different for females than for males."

"Master, I am not interested in learning about females." Pei Ke thought of the times he was nervous being around girls his own age. He wanted to meet them but didn't know quite how to go about it.

"Then you are not interested in learning about yourself."

Pei Ke started to protest, but Liu held up his hand and the student closed his mouth. Liu continued.

"You are trying to learn about only one-half of the Yin Yang concept. Remember your masculinity is only part of the Yin Yang concept. Within you as a male, there is a little bit of female and within every female, there is a little bit of male. You should be aware of it, for you will never understand your maleness until you understand your complimentary opposite."

"I am sorry Master. You are correct, of course."

"The book Simple Questions was written hundreds of years ago. It mentions differences that exist between the development of males and females. These differences are due in part to the development of the kidney energy. From the time a girl is born until she reaches approximately the age of seven, the kidney energy is building in her body. Her baby teeth fall out and become replaced by her permanent teeth. She will notice her hair grows longer and is more luxurious. By the time she reaches puberty, which is approximately the age of fourteen, her menstruation has started. This is the time she is able to conceive a child. When a woman reaches the age of twenty-one, her kidney energy peaks, her wisdom teeth come in, and her upward growth is finished. When she reaches the age of twenty-eight, she is at her maximum physical strength. At this time, she will accomplish more in life than at any other time. This kidney energy starts to decrease by the time she reaches thirty-five. She will then notice that her complexion changes and takes on a slightly darkened hue. Her hair begins to fall out. When she approaches the age of forty-two, her face takes on an even darker appearance and loses some of its sheen. Much to her dismay, her hair continues to fall out. She has far less stamina than in previous years. When a woman reaches forty-nine, her menstruation will begin to cease and she will no longer be able to conceive a child. These changes in age probably correspond to chemical and hormonal changes taking place in the woman's body. Not all the chemical and hormonal changes are pleasant. Notice that these stages in a woman's life are in multiples of seven years. Think of it as a seven-year itch and you will be able to remember it. That is the nature of being a woman."

"Master, what you describe is almost exactly what happened to my mother. As I look back, she went through some of the same changes you speak of, but I think the ages were maybe a little different. Perhaps a little earlier than what you indicated. Maybe diet had something to do with it; we didn't have a lot of food to eat and sometimes what we did have wasn't very good."

"Yes, you are correct. Diet plays an important role. In addition, the ages can be different because of the quality of the Primordial Qi and the Post Heaven Qi your mother had."

Pei Ke thought of his mother, of the way she somehow managed to find a bit of meat or something for him and his siblings, when all she had was a little rice. Before he had gone too far into his daydream, he realized Master Liu was still talking.

"Now that you know about the kidney energy and how it relates to females you need to know about how it relates to you. At the age of eight, a boy has an abundance of energy that helps his hair and teeth grow stronger. When a boy turns sixteen, he experiences a hormonal awakening and his sperm is able to successfully impregnate a woman. At twenty-four, the boy is now a man and his kidney energy reaches its peak. His bones are strong and growth is at its peak. At thirty-two, he feels physically fit. He will be most productive at this time of his life. His tendons and bones are at their strongest and the body is physically at its peak. When the man turns forty, the kidney energy weakens. His hair begins to fall out. His teeth no longer have their strength and start to fall out. At forty-eight, the face becomes a little darker with age spots. The remaining hair turns gray. At the age of fifty-six, his energy is weaker and his physical strength is noticeably weaker. By the time he reaches sixty-four, the teeth and hair are substantially affected. Note that the development of women is faster than the development of men"

"Master, you are much older than you look yet your teeth are good and your hair is still dark. What is your secret?"

"The cultivation of the Qi is the secret. Also, I avoid excesses, especially those things that deplete kidney energy."

"What depletes kidney energy?"

"Many things deplete kidney energy. Excessive sexual activity dampens the kidney Qi for men. Having a large number of children or especially difficult deliveries weakens the kidney energy in women. Kidney Qi can also be damaged from injuries to the back."

"Master, what is the result of not having the right amount of Qi in our kidneys?"

"The ancient doctors were good observers of nature, and the interaction of the various activities in our bodies. When kidney Qi is not correct, the result may be low back pain, knee pain, ankle pain, ringing in the ears, deafness, and loss of hair and or hair color."

"From what you have told me, Qi in its many forms and its development throughout our life is the only concept that is important in medicine."

"No, Qi is important, but many other concepts exist that you need to be aware of if you are to become a true doctor. You also need to know about the concept of Blood."

Pei Ke frowned.

"Isn't blood the red liquid flowing through our bodies, and it escapes when we get cut?"

"Yes and no. It is more than the liquid flowing through our bodies. The Blood comes from a complex interaction between the stomach, spleen, lungs, and heart. The stomach receives the food we eat. The food becomes processed into energy, and this energy is sent to the spleen, which transforms this into nutrition. It passes on to the lungs and then to the heart where it becomes Blood. Its essence, though, is in the spleen. Without Qi our bodies would be unable to go through this elaborate process. Thus, Qi and Blood are intermixed. In addition, we can think of Blood as a form of Qi."

"Master, I am thoroughly confused."

"Yes, it is a difficult concept initially to understand. For now think of Blood as a form of Qi that is Yin by nature, whereas basic Qi is Yang. Does that help?"

"I think so."

"Good. Now let us return to our discussion of the meridians. Doctors refer to these meridians as the Twelve Main or Classical Meridians. Some doctors include the Conception Vessel Meridian, which is on the front midline and the Governing Vessel Meridian, which is on the back midline as part of the Main or Classical Meridians. When they include these two meridians, they refer to the collection of meridians as the Fourteen Main or Classical Meridians.

"The Conception Vessel Meridian, which is Yin in nature, begins in the area of the anus at the acupuncture point Hui Yin, and runs up the front of the body to the acupuncture point Cheng Jiang, which is located in a depression in the groove below the lower lip. The Governing Vessel Meridian, which is Yang in nature, begins at the acupuncture point Cheng Jiang. This point is located between the tip of the tailbone and the center of the anus. This meridian travels upward along the spine to the top of the head and over the tip of the nose to the acupuncture point Yin Jiao, located on gums behind the upper lip.

"You need to make sure you do not become confused between the classification of the Twelve Meridians and the classification of the Fourteen Meridians. The Conception Vessel Meridian and the Governing Vessel Meridian are actually part of a classification called the Eight Extra Meridians, but are often added into the classification of the Twelve Basic Meridians because they are used quite often in treating imbalances."

"Master, what are the Eight Extra Meridians?"

"The Eight Extra Meridians are the Governing Vessel Meridian, Conception Vessel Meridian, Yang Heel Meridian, Yin Heel Meridian, Yang Linking Meridian, Yin Linking Meridian, and Belt Meridian, which is sometimes called Waist Meridian or Thoroughfare Meridian. One main difference between the Twelve Main Meridians and the Eight Extra Meridians is that none of the eight are associated with an internal organ. If you remember, the Lung Meridian is associated with the lungs, Large Intestine Meridian is associated with the large intestine organ, and so on.

"With the exception of the Governing Vessel Meridian and the Conception Vessel Meridian, these meridians do not have their own acupuncture points; they share the acupuncture points of other meridians.

"Think of these Eight Extra Meridians as pathways that join, store, and regulate the internal energy and blood in our body. You can also think of the Eight Extra Meridians as reservoirs or safety nets absorbing energy directly from the Twelve Main Meridians or transferring energy back to the Twelve Main Meridians when needed."

"Master, how does it happen that these meridians absorb the energy of the Main Meridians?

"The subject is a little advanced for you now. The answer will only be confusing."

In a somewhat hesitant voice, Pei Ke asked, "Are there any more meridians?"

"Yes, in addition to the Main Meridians, Connecting Meridians, and Eight Extra Meridians there are Internal Meridians and Muscle Meridians. The Internal Meridians are actually branches from the Main Meridians that disperse the energy to the applicable organs, complimentary opposite organs, and other parts of the body. Do you understand?"

"No, it is too confusing."

"Here is an example. The Small Intestine Meridian starts at the outside cuticle of the little finger, travels up the arm to the shoulder and scapula, over to the spine and up the neck to the face and ear. This is the main pathway of the meridian, and it is along this pathway where the acupuncture points are located. From what I have just described, it would seem the Small Intestine Meridian, as you now visualize it, does not connect with the small intestine.

"Since each Main Meridian is associated with an organ, there has to be some connection to the organ. In the case of the small intestine, a pathway branches off the Small Intestine Meridian in the area of the collar bone. The branch has no acupuncture points. It goes from the collar bone inside the body to the heart, diaphragm, stomach, and finally to the small intestine itself. This is the reason you can stimulate an acupuncture point on the hand and actually affect the small intestine. Do you understand?"

"Yes, that helps, but I will need to spend more time thinking about it."

"The Muscle Meridians are nothing more than a series of muscles connected energetically. They follow in close proximity to the Twelve Main Meridians. There are no acupuncture points on the Muscle Meridians."

"What do they do if they are not really connected to anything?"

Liu looked at his student.

"You have a good question. What I am about to tell you is only my opinion, and not the opinion of others. Remember I told you about the energy in our bodies being stimulated by the food we eat, the water we drink, the air we breathe, and the exercise we do?"

"Yes, Master."

"I believe when we do exercises like Tai Chi Chuan and Qi Gong, we are stimulating the energy along the Muscle Meridians which in turn stimulates the energy of the Main Meridians."

"But how is this done?"

"The Muscle Meridian pathway has a connection with the Main Meridian at different points. As an example, the Heart Meridian starts at the chest and runs down the arm to the little finger. The Heart Muscle Meridian also starts in the chest and runs down the arm to the little finger. When you visualize the two together, where the segments of the various muscles of the Heart Muscle Meridian join together are also locations where there are acupuncture points on the Heart Meridian."

"Master?"

Liu held up his hand.

"Enough, you need to think about what I have told you. Your questions will be answered later. We are nearing the village. Take this message to Mr. Li who is the herbalist here. You can find him on White Lotus Street next to the meat market. When you are finished with him, meet me at the teahouse at the north end of the village."

"How will I be able to find the teahouse?"

"There is only one teahouse in the village. Mr. Wang owns it. Ask the herbalist. Now go and don't dally."

# CHAPTER FOUR

"Master Liu, this is a pleasant surprise! It is my honor to have you come."

Liu instantly recognized the voice as Wang walked toward Liu's table. Wang was dressed in a long, gray silk robe, quite out of place for a working owner at a teahouse. The robe was in sharp contrast to the bright colors of his surroundings. Wang's presence was therefore always known. He kept his collar buttoned tightly but his sleeves open, and he kept his hands inserted into the opposite sleeves. Few knew Wang kept a dagger up one sleeve and a razor-sharp throwing dart up the other. Liu had never asked Wang about the weapons, but he knew Wang had them. He guessed that someone in Wang's position could make enemies, and it was wise to be prepared for the worst.

Liu had not seen Wang since the man's last visit to the temple to make one of his generous offerings. Wang's walk was steadier; the leg injury he had asked Liu to treat must have healed. Wang told Liu he had fallen, but Liu knew from the way Wang walked that the injury had come from a blow or kick to the knee area. Wang was lucky to have come away with just a bruise. An attack to that area of the knee could permanently cripple a person.

"I am honored to have such a noble person come to my humble business," said Wang as he bowed to Liu.

Liu returned the bow. Wang turned and waved to one of the girls to bring some tea. The girls were all dressed alike in pink silk clothes resembling custom-made uniforms.

"I presume some green tea would be to your liking?" said Wang. "I have some very special tea that has come my way. Have you eaten, Master?"

Yes, thank you, I would like some tea. Someone will join me shortly. After he comes would you be so kind as to prepare us some tofu, vegetables, and rice?"

"Of course. It is quite late in the day. Will you be returning to the temple, or do you need a place to stay for the night?"

"We would like to stay here in the village for the night. Do you know where there are suitable accommodations?"

"We have guest accommodations here in the back." He motioned to a hallway leading away from the area where Liu sat. "You are welcome to stay as long as you wish."

"Thank you, Wang. We will only be staying the evening. How are your wife and your oldest son?"

"Thanks to you, they are both fine. Please excuse me for a moment, I must see to your meal and room. We will talk later."

As Wang walked across the room, the two men who had been following Liu entered and took seats nearby. Neither one of them stared at Liu, but occasionally they would look and make a gesture in his direction as if they were contemplating some action. Liu sipped his tea and mentally agreed with Wang. The tea was indeed of superior quality.

As Liu quietly sipped his tea, Pei Ke entered through the main door. Besides Liu and the girls in pink, the only other people who noticed his student enter the teahouse were the two men sitting at the table.

Pei Ke walked over to where Liu was sitting. Liu motioned for him to take a seat. "Master, I took the message to the herbalist as you instructed. He said he would take care of sending the herbs to Master Ma. What are the herbs for?"

"Master Ma has asthma and the herbs are to help him with his breathing."

"The herbalist explained some things about herbs. When I told him I was one of your students, he looked very surprised."

"What did he say?"

"He said he didn't know you were taking any more students."

"What did he tell you about herbs?"

"He indicated some herbs are for warming, others are for cooling, tonifying, dispersing, and expectorating. He told me exactly what you told me. Before giving herbs to the patient, you must do a differential diagnosis taking into consideration all the signs and symptoms. He didn't quite say it the same way you said it, but after I thought about it, I understood that he had used different words to express the same meaning."

"I cannot stress enough the importance of taking not only the pulses when making a diagnosis but also evaluating the overall condition of the patient. The four diagnostic protocols are critical," said Liu. Liu motioned toward the tea pot. Pei Ke nodded and poured himself some tea.

"When my parents went to the Chinese doctor, he diagnosed their problems first," Pei Ke said. "Then he would do either acupuncture or a combination of acupuncture and herbal formulas. I often saw the doctor go into another room where he kept a wall cabinet with hundreds of drawers. At first, I thought the cabinet contained only dried herbs, but later I learned that in addition to different herbs, the doctor had various animal parts and earthly substances.

"He usually wanted my parents to take the herbs for a specific number of days. Each day's herbs were wrapped in rice paper and tied with a string. Each day they unwrapped the packet and put the herbs into two cups of water. They then boiled and simmered the concoction until it was reduced to a cup of concentrated tea. They let it cool and then drank it. It must have tasted terrible because they made faces while drinking the liquid. The doctor always included with each packet little pieces of plum candy to help reduce the terrible taste."

"Did the herbalist tell you why there are so many different ingredients in the formulas?"

"No, Master."

"Well, first of all, Chinese herbal formulas are seldom, if ever, prescribed as a single substance. Multiple herbs, minerals and animal parts are used for each formula. Each component in the formula has a specific function. As an example, the formula for Master Ma is composed of many different items, one of which is Ma Huang. Ma Huang is used because it opens up the lungs. It is the herb of choice for many lung problems. If I were to leave this herb out of the formula, he would not experience the same results."

"Master, are acupuncture and Chinese herbal formulas the only two ways to help Master Ma?"

"Master Ma could practice Qi Gong and Tai Chi Chuan to build up his internal energy, especially his kidney Qi. It is the kidney and lung Qi in Master Ma that is causing him to have his asthma. Both Qi Gong and Tai Chi Chuan are excellent ways to enhance this internal energy."

"Why doesn't Master Ma do these exercises?"

"I mentioned it to him on numerous occasions but he always indicated he was too busy with activities in the temple. Each of us makes decisions based on the information we have available at the time and the accumulation of previous experience. His previous experience prevented him from making a good decision."

"Master, I..."

"Here comes Mr. Wang with our food."

"Master Liu, I have prepared a special meal for you," Wang said. "We used the finest ingredients. I trust you will find them to your liking."

Liu Introduced Pei Ke to Wang and Pei Ke bowed in respect. Wang and a serving girl placed four dishes on Liu's table. The main staple as usual was long grain white rice. The second dish had tofu sprinkled with finely chopped green onions, topped with a dark soy sauce and sesame seed oil. The plate of mixed vegetables included white radish, dark mushrooms, bamboo shoots, and water chestnuts. The last dish was steamed baby Bok Choi topped with a slightly sweet plum sauce and sesame seed oil. The color of the vegetables, the aroma and the taste gave the meal the perfect balance of Yin and Yang

"Master, enjoy the meal," Wang said. He turned and hurried across the room to his vantage point by the door.

Liu and Pei Ke ate in silence for a few minutes. Liu was about to relate more information about treating patients when Pei Ke interrupted him.

"Master."

"Yes."

"This food is very good. Wang is an outstanding cook. Have you eaten here before?"

"No, this is the first time, but I have heard of his skill. Would you like to know more about how the food is prepared?"

"No, Master. I have no interest in being a cook."

"Do you have an interest in learning all the underlying concepts of the universal energy?"

"Of course, Master. That is why I want to be with you. I want to learn everything you know and more."

"Pei Ke, go invite Wang to join us."

"Yes, Master."

As Pei Ke walked across the room, Liu had the uneasy feeling of a disruption in the balance of Yin and Yang. He'd had the same feeling when his father had passed away many years earlier, like a void or imbalance in the universal energy. It meant conflict and he knew from experience that conflicts had a way of resolving themselves. The important thing was how they became resolved. One resolution might lead to another conflict, which would then need a second resolution.

"Master Liu, is there something wrong with the food?" Wang asked.

"No," said Liu. "The food is superb. It is true what others have said about your skill. If you have a moment, however, would you be so kind as to explain to Pei Ke some of the underlying concepts of how you prepare the food?"

"I didn't know your student had an interest in cooking."

"Actually, I would also like to learn more about cooking, and especially how you do it so well."

"Master, you are so kind," said Wang. "You already know the essence of cooking. There is nothing more I can tell you."

Pei Ke listened as the two men talked.

He never knew Liu could cook. It was amazing what this old master seems to know. Not only was he a great master of martial arts, literature, and medicine, but he also knew and studied the great philosophical words, wrote poetry, painted, and practiced calligraphy. It would be impossible to learn all that he knew. Pei Ke worried that it might be a hopeless and futile endeavor to even think he could be as great as the master.

"There is always something to learn," said Liu. "Please tell us something about your skill."

Liu motioned for Wang to sit. One of the serving girls immediately came to the table with a cup, poured the tea for Wang and refilled the other cups. Wang acknowledged the service and the girl seemed pleased that Wang would acknowledge such a simple action on her part.

"There really isn't anything to tell." Wang smiled and looked down at his folded arms.

"We have known each other for some time," Liu said. "We need not remain on a formal basis with each other. Please share with us some of the secrets."

"What would you like to know?" Wang asked. He poured more tea for Liu and motioned for the serving girl to bring another pot.

"This tea is, as you said, excellent. Where did you get it?"

"If we are going to talk tea, it is important that you know something about tea," Wang said.

"Please, enlighten us," Master Liu said.

Wang bowed his head.

"All the references to tea deal with the processing of the tea leaves," he said. "Though there is only one tea plant, there are many different ways of fermenting the tea leaves which produce a variety of flavors. Tea fermentation is classified into five basic categories: green tea, which you are drinking now, black tea, brick tea, tea with scented flowers and the strong tasting Oolong tea.

"Some say the drinking of tea is a tradition dating back 4,500 years. Of course, I don't know if that is quite true, but history indicates the tradition is quite old.

"In the Song dynasty, Liu You, who came to be known as the Tea Sage, wrote a detailed description in the Tea Scripture detailing the method of planting tea, the process of harvesting, and the preparing and brewing of tea leaves. Tea along with fuel, rice, oil, salt, soy sauce, and vinegar are often referred to as the basics of life.

"Good teas come from all over this land, but some of the finest teas are grown at altitudes above three thousand feet. The difference between green tea and black or Oolong tea is that the tea leaves have gone through different stages of a fermentation process. The tea you are drinking now is a mixture of Huang Shan Mao Feng green tea from Huang Shan in An Hui,

Du Yun Mao Jian tea from Du Yun Shan and Wu Yi Rock Tea from Wu Yi Shan. To this blend, I add an herb that Master Liu knows, called Bai He and some Chrysanthemum blossoms. You will only find my special blend at this teahouse."

Liu nodded approvingly.

"Tell us about all these delicious dishes and how you learned to prepare them so well." Liu drank deeply from his cup, enjoying the aroma of the tea.

"There is a legend about food preparation," said Wang. "The great mystical figure Fu Shi was the first person to teach the benefits of cooking. His teachings were disseminated throughout the four corners of our country. However, each area developed the basics a little differently depending on the people living in that area, what the land would grow, and what resources were available. For example, wheat is grown mostly north of the great Yangzi River and so most people there eat noodles, while rice is the predominant grain grown south of the river. In the south, near the ocean, the diet is composed mostly of seafood. In the north people eat more pork. In Sichuan and Hunan provinces, the people use more hot peppers in their cooking."

He glanced around the tearoom. Several men had taken a table by the window.

"Master, let me finish later, I need to make sure my guests have been taken care of."

Wang got up and left the table and Liu turned to Pei Ke. "I want you to take this note back to the herbalist. Do not waste time. I want you back soon. You can eat later."

"Yes, Master." Pei Ke got up immediately from the table and walked toward the door. He kept his face straight until he was out of the teahouse, but then he scowled. His food would be cold when he returned, if there was any left at all. Why would Teacher send him out just when he started to eat?

Pei Ke turned left from the teahouse and headed down North Star Street toward the herbalist. He had walked this route not more than an hour earlier. He decided at the next corner to take a different route to his destination. On his first walk to the herbalist, he had seen many vendors selling everything from carved jade to food. On this second trip he again moved quickly, but he took in everything possible, for he had never seen so many people in one area selling and buying. It was almost overpowering. If only he had some money so he could buy some things. He hoped one day he would be rich enough to enjoy everything he had missed in his childhood.

On his first trip to the herbalist he had the uneasy feeling that someone was watching him. If someone was following him, they would expect him to take the same route. Instead of continuing down North Star Street, he turned at the next street.

———————

Liu noticed that the two men sitting across the room got up when Pei Ke left the teahouse. Liu rose from his chair and started to move toward the door when Wang motioned for him to return to his seat. As their eyes met, Liu knew the situation was well under control. Wang was a martial artist like Liu and knew almost everyone in the area who practiced any type of martial arts. Wang went immediately to the back and whispered to one of the helpers in the kitchen. When Wang returned to the dining area, he nodded to Liu and smiled. Liu sat down at his table, but was still concerned for the safety of his student. Pei Ke would be no match for any skilled martial artist.

# CHAPTER FIVE

"Pei Ke, you are back so soon. Was the herbalist there?"

"Yes, Master."

"Did you give him the note?"

"Yes, Master. He said he would handle it."

"Did he say anything else?"

"No, but he gave me a funny look and said he would take care of everything. I didn't think you would want me to bother him with questions, so I told him you needed me back at the teahouse. He just nodded and I left."

"What was he doing when you arrived? Did he appear very busy?"

"He was mixing some herbs. There were some pots on his stove and he was writing something in one of his books. He had enough prescriptions to fill to keep him busy for awhile."

"Was there anyone in the shop helping him?"

"I didn't see anyone except the herbalist, but I heard noises in the back of the shop. And a couple of women were outside talking; I guess they were waiting for their herbs to be concocted."

Liu looked up and saw Wang talking with one of his kitchen staff. Wang turned and faced Liu and smiled. Liu felt better.

Before the master could ask him anymore questions or send him on another errand, Pei Ke quickly helped himself to the remaining food. The master did not seem to notice his haste, though Pei Ke thought he probably did.

"I have known that herbalist for many years," said Liu. "He is a very good martial artist, though few know it. His father and my father trained together for many years when they were young. They studied from some of the same teachers. Actually, because of the close relationship, our family helped him get started in his business."

"Why don't people know the truth about him?" Pei Ke said, barely swallowing his food before the question slipped out.

"He does not let many people know this because he wants to keep a certain image. As you know, many people look down on martial artists as being crude, uneducated, and second-class individuals.

"He knows many martial artists within the brotherhood. It is a very close collection of individuals, each with their own specialty, drawn together in mutual friendship. Many have a family martial arts lineage, where only members of the family know that particular martial art. Someday you will meet some of them."

"Master, why do people look down on martial artists?" asked Pei Ke. He picked up the teapot and refilled both their cups. The master looked at him closely before shaking his head.

"I don't have a good answer for you. It just seems that in our culture, things of the mind take precedent over things of the body. Of course this is an unbalanced situation on either side and a misrepresentation of what we do. When there is excess anywhere there is a health problem. Physical activities of the body, like martial arts, affect activities of the mind, and activities of the mind influence activities of the body.

"Those people who do physical exercise like martial arts usually feel much better than those who do not exercise at all. In Tai Chi Chuan, Hsing-Yi Chuan, and Pa Kua Chang, it is the mind that has a lot to do with the production of internal energy. The mind and body both need to be in balance. That is why it is important for you to be good in martial arts, calligraphy, medicine, literature, and painting. The underlying principles of all these disciplines are the same. The key is balance."

"I will be studying something for the rest of my life," Pei Ke muttered.

"Did you not listen to what I said at the temple when you chose this path?" Master Liu said. Pei Ke looked at his bowl in embarrassment but did not say anything.

"Now," Master Liu said, sipping his tea, "tell me exactly the year, day, and time you were born."

Pei Ke looked up, obviously grateful to be discussing something other than his undisciplined thoughts, but he also looked slightly dismayed.

"I don't know exactly, Master, but I think I was born in the late 1800's."

"You are not sure?"

"No, Master. My father had a shop in the village. When he came home for the evening, he tended to the fields behind the house. Then he took care of the animals. He worked until dark and then did more work in the little hut where we lived. My mother worked as a seamstress. She took in work while staying home to take care of us children. Neither of them was educated and no birth records were kept of when I was born. I asked about my birthday once. My parents spent some time trying to remember different events and seasons and told me it was probably 1890."

"Then you were born in the year of the monkey."

"Is that significant to you, Master?"

"No. In itself it means nothing. But you are young. If you choose, you will be able to learn more about it than I know."

"About what, Master?"

Master Liu leaned back, his eyes passing unnoticed on the other patrons of the teahouse.

"From an astrological point of view, the year of your birth means a lot. In the order of the Chinese Zodiac, monkey is ninth. It follows those born in the year of the sheep and precedes those born in the year of the rooster."

"Master, I know there are others, like snake and horse. What is the actual order of all the astrological animals?"

"The correct order is rat, ox, tiger, rabbit, dragon, snake, horse, sheep, monkey, rooster, dog, and pig.

"Those that were born in the year of the monkey tend to have common characteristics of being intelligent, witty, ambitious, successful, agile and lively. They are usually amusing, self centered, and a little devious. In marriage, they are most compatible with someone born either in the year of the dragon or in the year of the rat. The dragon is charismatic, extroverted, optimistic, and loyal. The rat is clever, astute, daring, hard working, flexible and active."

"In Chinese astrology there are the Twelve Earthly Branches of the year, and Ten Heavenly Stems. Taken together they tell a lot about a person."

"In addition each animal is either Yin or Yang. The Yang animals are rat, tiger, dragon, horse, monkey, and dog. The Yin animals are ox, rabbit, snake, sheep, rooster, and pig. In the Twelve Earthly Branches, the year of the monkey is always going to be Metal. However, in the Ten Heavenly Stems, it is determined that you can be any one of the Five Elements depending on the year you were born."

"Which one am I?"

"It becomes very complicated. Do you know what day and time you were born?"

"No, Master. My mother said I was born late at night, in the early summer just after the yearly spring rains and before the summer heat.

"According to the philosophical concept of the Five Elements, Metal, Water, Wood, Fire, and Earth form the essential structure of all things living. Each animal has a sixty-year cycle governed or ruled by a different element. There are twelve animals and five elements. The combinations change in sequence of the flow of the two factors. In addition to this combination, there are twelve two-hour periods. The rat is associated with the eleventh hour in the evening to the first hour in the morning. The ox is associated with the first hour in the morning to the third hour in the morning, and so on.

"If you remember, earlier I told you that in Chinese medicine, it is possible to determine a person's constitutional make up by knowing the day and time of the birth. This will determine the tendency one has towards a constitutional imbalance. Once this is known, it is then possible to treat the patient constitutionally. This knowledge is valuable when you have a patient whom you have difficulty diagnosing because the signs and symptoms and your differential diagnosis are not helpful.

"Many good physicians refer to a book listing all the combinations of animals, elements, and time. These books usually have birth dates starting many years before and go forward to time in the future. Therefore, if one was born seventy years ago, the doctor is able to look up the constitution of this person. Thus for each child born, the basic constitution of that child is already known at birth."

"My mother's sister was there when I was born. She may have more information on the day and time. It just did not seem important to them."

"Most people in general do not pay attention to their exact birthday. Is your aunt still alive?"

"As far as I know. I don't even remember what she looks like. She and her husband live east of here by the coast. Mother told me my uncle was a fisherman, and he spent most of his time at sea. Like us, they were poor and probably never traveled too far from their home."

"If you ever see your aunt again, ask her about your birth, and I will share with you some of the information relevant to your birthday."

The master stood up.

"While you were at the herbalist I spoke with Wang. His wife Wang Yi is not feeling well and his youngest son has a shoulder injury. It is appropriate for us to help them. This will be a good learning experience for you."

"Yes, Master," Pei Ke said, also rising.

"They are waiting for us."

"Yes, Master. While we walk, may I ask you one more question?"

He always has only one question, thought Liu. He wondered what Pei Ke had in mind next. Together, they left the tearoom and Liu nodded for his student to continue.

"Master, you mentioned previously that there is tonification and dispersion of energy. How do you do this?"

"There are many techniques for tonifying and dispersing energy, and the benefits the patient receives depend on the level of expertise of the practitioner. For example, a newly trained practitioner will probably only be concerned with accurately locating the points and acquiring the stimulation of energy. A practitioner who is more experienced may want to tonify and disperse the energy by either rapid or slow insertion depending on the condition. An advanced practitioner knows a number of different ways to stimulate the energy. It depends on whether the patient is male or female, which side of the body is affected, the direction of energy flow, and so on. The most important thing is to understand what causes the imbalance and how to harmonize the imbalance."

"Master, with so many different and contradictory ways to stimulate the energy, how does one get it right?"

"I can make it simpler for you. You want to tonify the energy when there is a deficiency and you want to disperse the energy when there is an excess. In general, a deficient condition is a weakness and the energy needs strengthening. An excess condition indicates an underlying pathogenic condition, or an overactive physiological condition. Here is an example: a cold, withdrawn, weak, depressed, passive condition in general is considered a deficiency; while a hot, expansive, strong, energetic, outward situation may be an excess. We strive to obtain a balanced position. Of the different methods of tonification and dispersion, I prefer the angle of insertion method for most of my treatments. I would utilize the other methods when the situation warrants their use."

"Why do you prefer the angle of insertion method?"

"It is complicated, but if you listen carefully you will understand," Liu said. "As I indicated before, energy flows along predetermined pathways. The Yin meridians of the leg flow along the inside of the leg and ascend from the toes toward the trunk of the body. The Yang meridians of the leg descend from the trunk of the body to the feet. Think of the flow as a major road and all the travelers can only go in one direction. Minor roads join the major road, but they join at an angle in the direction of flow. The new travelers flow along and merge into the flow of traffic. Thus, the needle is inserted in the direction the flow is going to tonify the energy. If the needle insertion is done in the opposite direction, or against the flow, then some of the energy will leave, or disperse.

"The angle of insertion is important, and this is where the expertise of the practitioner is important. The needle can be inserted perpendicular to the point, which balances the energy. The practitioner does not want to increase or deplete too much energy. He only wants to unblock what is blocked and get the energy to move along the pathway. The needle can be inserted at an oblique angle, which will give more tonification or dispersion. The needle can also be inserted horizontally, which maximizes the amount of stimulation. The practitioner needs to increase the energy or reduce the energy based on the signs and symptoms and his differential diagnosis.

"If a lot of energy needs to be affected, the angle from the perpendicular will be large, otherwise, the angle must be small. Too much tonification may cause an adverse effect, as can too much dispersion. When you are using the tonification and dispersion in this manner, you need to be sure the patient is comfortable and healthy.

"One can also use combinations of the methods I've described. Only a practitioner well versed in acupuncture should use combinations to prevent too much tonification or dispersion."

"Master, is it always necessary to tonify or disperse?"

"Since our health issues are due to an imbalance of energy—either too much or too little—then tonification and dispersion are usually appropriate. Some practitioners only insert the needle and do neither tonification nor dispersion. It is believed that once De Qi, or the arrival of the energy, has taken place no further manipulation is necessary."

"What does the patient actually feel?"

Liu stopped walking as he thought of an appropriate answer. There was silence as Liu turned to Pei Ke.

"Acupuncture is quite painless. In many instances, the patient feels nothing on needle insertion. After needle insertion, the patient will feel De Qi, which is the arrival of the energy. It is mentioned in the ancient book Miraculous Pivot that the beneficial effects of the acupuncture treatment will not happen unless the De Qi effect is felt by the patient. Even today, most practitioners believe the arrival of the energy is vital for the patient's improvement. There is some truth to that; however, I believe while it is important to get this feeling, the treatment is not a failure if the patient does not feel it."

"Master, what does the De Qi effect feel like?"

"The patient and the doctor will both feel something, though what they feel is different. The patient can feel a slight soreness, heaviness, distension, or numbness in close proximity to the acupuncture point. In some cases, the patient will feel energy moving along the pathway of the meridian. It feels strange, but does not hurt. Those who have had acupuncture before will actually help you by telling you when the energy has arrived. They actually look forward to this effect for they know they will be better after the treatment.

"The practitioner can feel something just as the patient feels something. He will feel a slight pulling sensation. In the book Lyrics of Standard Profundities, it suggests that the feeling of De Qi is similar to the feeling of a fish biting on a hook. In many instances, you will also see the muscles twitch around the site of the needle. Again, it should not be painful nor uncomfortable for the patient. Usually they feel very relaxed and peaceful. Many times they will comment that they have not felt this relaxed in a long time. Once they feel this relaxation they look forward to their next visit."

Liu looked around for Wang's residence and motioned for them to continue walking. It was getting dark and they could hear insects and night birds beginning their aural interplay.

"Master. Just one more question. How can you use Qi Gong to stimulate the energy?"

Liu chuckled.

"You may be a student, Pei Ke," Liu said, "but you are a master of turning one question into many."

Pei Ke blushed and hoped the master could not tell, but Liu said nothing else about it and proceeded to answer the question.

"You can tonify or disperse energy by focusing on your thoughts or you can affect the energy with your breathing pattern. These techniques are some of the highest levels of practice, and should only be done by an experienced practitioner of both acupuncture and Qi Gong. I will provide a more satisfactory answer when such an answer will mean more to you."

Pei Ke nodded and hesitated to ask his next question, but before he knew it, he had asked it anyway.

"Master, how long do we leave the needles in the patient?" He was so fascinated and interested, he could not seem to control himself.

"There are different theories as to how long the needles should be retained," Liu said, pausing outside Wang's home. "The most important factor is whether or not the acupuncture point has been located correctly. If located correctly, the patient will feel the arrival of energy. As I just mentioned this could feel like a distention, an achy feeling, tingling sensation, or a slight electrical sensation. Some practitioners think that once this is accomplished, the needles can be immediately removed, as the energy is no longer unbalanced. Most practitioners feel that the needles should be left in for fifteen to twenty minutes for the patient to get the maximum benefit. In addition, some teachers feel the needles need to be stimulated occasionally during the treatment process by either tonifying or dispersing more of the energy. How much you do depends on what the patient tells you and your experience in this particular type of problem. You must think about the manner in which you are dispersing the energy. As indicated before, I like to use the slanting insertion method of tonification or dispersion since I can control the amount of energy I add or take away. However, since the needle is continuously adding or taking away energy as long as I leave the needle in the patient, I need to be careful not to overdo the treatment process."

"When I went with my parents to the doctor, he had many different types of needles. Why are there so many different types of needles?"

"Each type of needle is used for a specific purpose. There are nine classical types of needles. Many of these needles are not commonly used today, but were used in ancient times for specific uses. The basic needles we use today are plum blossom needles, tri-edged needles, and thin needles.

Plum blossom needles have five to seven equally spaced needles bundled together to form a head on a flexible bamboo stick. The needles are lightly tapped on the skin with a whipping motion to cause the skin to become red. This technique is often used on children. It will cause the expelling of heat from the body at the site of tapping. The plum blossom needles are used to treat diseases along the pathway of the meridians or specific conditions that cause numbness and tingling. You must be very careful not to use these needles again without thoroughly cleaning them, to prevent other patients from contracting an infection. Strict sterilization techniques must be followed.

"A tri-edged needle is used to get heat out of the body. It causes bleeding at a specific acupuncture point to release the heat or congestion. A good example would be to use the Shao Shang point located at the outside cuticle of the thumb to reduce heat in the throat or lungs. Heat in the lungs causes a sore throat. I have used this technique numerous times on myself to get rid of a sore throat.

"Thin needles are used for general acupuncture to tonify or disperse the energy. These are now the most commonly used needles. In ancient times, there were needles to do cutting and other techniques but these are not a part of today's general practice. You only need to be proficient with these three for now. I will show you how to use them when the time is appropriate."

"Master, you said that sterilization was very important. How do you clean your needles?"

"In ancient times there was no knowledge that once a needle was used it should not be re-used until it was cleaned. Today we understand that there is a need to clean the needles. To prepare the needle for the next patient I prefer to subject the needle to intense heat before each use. I put the needle into a wok and place the wok on an intense fire for a few minutes. Sometimes I hold the needle into a hot flame. In either case, I always cool the needle and use it immediately after being cooled."

"Master, what is…?"

"Pei Ke, we are here to treat Mrs. Wang and her son, not to stand outside their door. You may ask one last question."

"Master, is it possible to hurt a patient with acupuncture?"

"It takes years of study and training under the guidance of a master acupuncturist to become an acupuncturist. If acupuncture is done correctly, there are virtually no side effects. The problem we have today is that many only study for a short period of time before practicing on patients. These people make me nervous. They trained in another field and want to use this art of acupuncture because they know of its benefits, but do not want to do the full training. An example would be those who practice muscle and bone manipulation. Manipulation techniques are their full-time professions. They learn a little acupuncture and call themselves experts.

"They usually travel to another town, do one or two weeks of training, and return home with some books. These people can actually do harm. They can either injure the patient or they can do the technique wrong. In either case, the patient does not get well or the symptoms become worse. The best advice to people is to thoroughly investigate the training of the practitioner before going for acupuncture treatments. The patient should ask questions such as where was the practitioner trained? Did he practice under the supervision of a master acupuncturist? How long was his acupuncture training? Was there advanced acupuncture training? How many years was the doctor in acupuncture training before he started to do acupuncture? Usually it takes four or more years of dedicated full time study under a master acupuncturist before you are qualified to treat patients. One should also inquire if acupuncture is his full time profession or just a sideline to his other work? Do you want a fully trained individual or an amateur doing the treatments? These same questions apply to all areas of Chinese Medicine and martial arts."

As they entered Wang's home, Pei Ke took a deep breath, overwhelmed by what he needed to know to become a truly exceptional doctor.

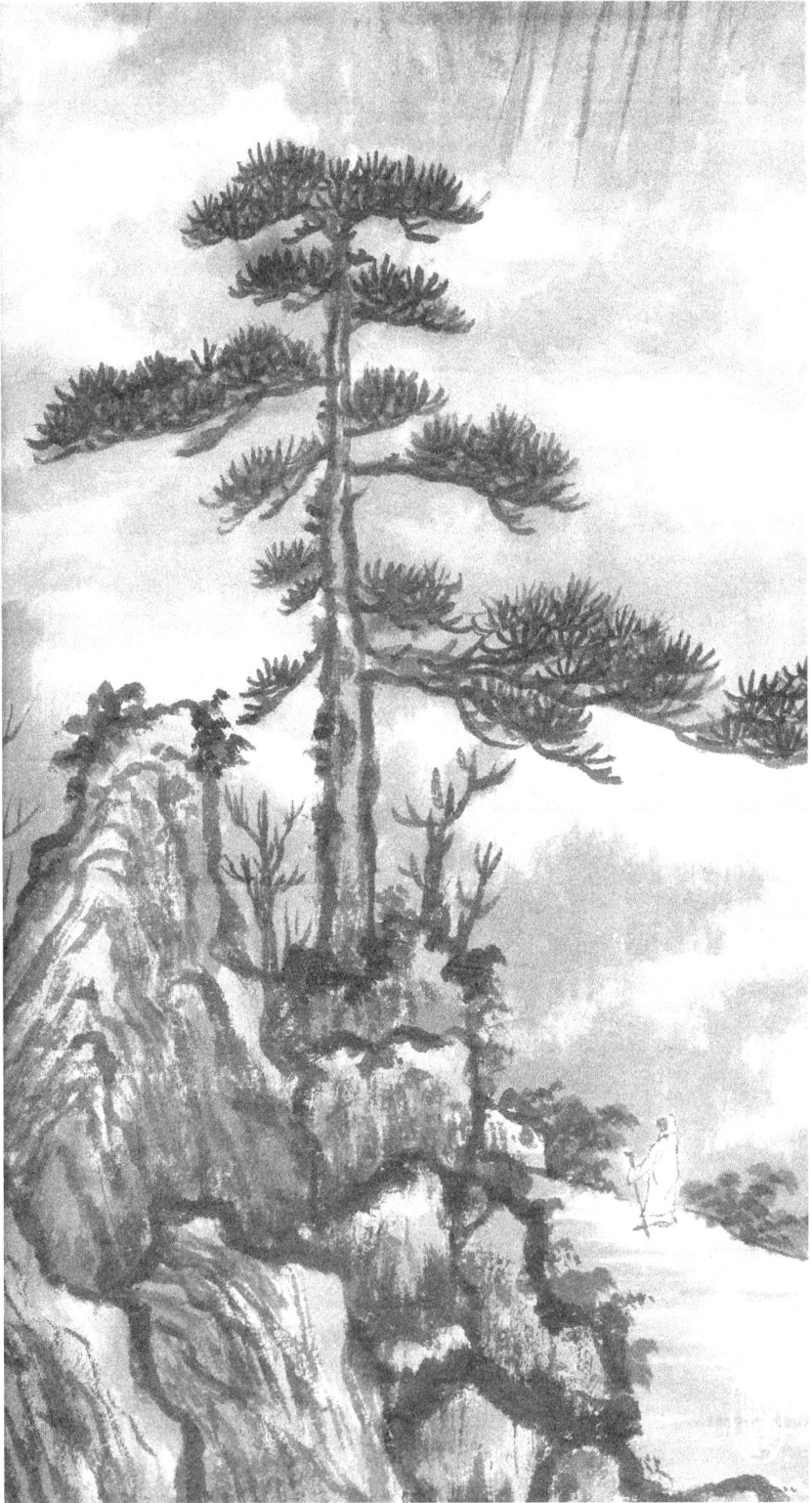

# CHAPTER SIX

"Mrs. Wang, how are you? The last time we spoke was at the temple when you came to make an offering. Thank you for your generosity."

"Please come in. It is a pleasure to see you again."

Liu and Pei Ke entered into the Wang's quarters. Liu introduced Pei Ke to Mrs. Wang. Pei Ke bowed low in respect.

"We are fine, Master Liu," Mrs. Wang said, "except for some occasional health problems. We are blessed. Many have problems much worse than mine, so I do not complain too much." Her eyes glittered slyly. "Of course at my age, I voice an occasional complaint so that everyone knows I am still here."

"Your husband has graciously allowed me and my student to stay this evening. While we are here, is there anything I can do for you?"

"You have helped us so much in the past and you have never asked for anything in return. It is I who should be helping you. Please take a seat."

Liu and Pei Ke sat down where Mrs. Wang indicated. She took a seat close by Liu's left side and Pei Ke sat to the master's right.

"You and your husband have always been kind and generous benefactors to the temple. If it were not for you two, we would not be able to help others. Your husband suggested I see if there is anything I can do for you while I am here. You mentioned occasional health problems."

"Yes, I seem to have a lot of headaches these last four months and our son has hurt his right shoulder. Do you think you can help? And of course I am getting fat."

"Would you mind if Pei Ke watches while I attend to you? He is a student of mine and he wants to learn about medicine."

Mrs. Wang looked at the young man for a few moments. "Pei Ke, do you really want to be a doctor like Master Liu?"

"Yes, Mrs. Wang," answered Pei Ke. "I will learn as much as Master Liu will teach me."

"You probably don't realize it but Master Liu is one of the most accomplished martial artists and healers I have ever known. You are lucky to have him as a teacher. We have come to trust Master Liu. It is a trust he has earned and never violated. I know whatever I tell Master Liu stays with Master Liu and is not divulged to anyone. Watch, learn, and absorb as much as you can, for you may never get another chance like this."

A chill went through Pei Ke as Mrs. Wang spoke. He sensed she was conveying more than one message. He could feel her penetrating eyes sizing him up for the second time.

"Pei Ke."

"Yes, Master."

"I want you to pay attention. Watch and listen, and do not ask any questions. I am sure you will find time to ask them later."

"Yes, Master."

"Mrs. Wang, can you tell me how long you have had these headaches?"

"About four months now. They are getting increasingly worse."

"Do you know why and how the headaches started?"

"No, but they are very debilitating. When I get one, my eyes hurt and my vision is somewhat blurred."

"Do you have the headaches occasionally or do you have them every day?"

"No, I don't have them every day, but maybe three to four times a week."

"Does the headache start at any particular time of the day or night?"

"Sometimes I wake up at the normal time in the morning with a headache, and sometimes the headache wakes me up in the middle of the night." Mrs. Wang shifted in her chair as if she could feel the headache at that moment.

"At approximately what time does it wake you at night?"

"Maybe one o'clock in the morning. If it wakes me up, it usually is so intense I cannot go back to sleep. When that happens I just get up."

"How long does the headache last and does it change in severity?"

"Often when I get them, I have a bitter taste in my mouth. After having something to eat, they usually go away by midday. Sometimes it will go away quickly, but other times it will disappear gradually; however, it is usually a throbbing-type headache. It feels like something is pounding on the inside of my head."

"Is the headache always on the side of your head or does it change places."

"It is usually on the right side, but it has also been on the left side." She smiled. "I know I am not much help, but this is how it happens. Usually, the headache goes away, but today the headache has been there since I got up this morning."

"You are doing fine, Mrs. Wang. Did your grandparents, parents, brothers, or sisters ever indicate that they had this type of a headache?"

"I don't think so. My mother had occasional headaches, but not like this. Her headaches were usually at her time of the month. They would be so bad she would have to go to bed and sometimes she would just lie in bed and moan for a day or so. When this happened I had to care for the family, so I remember it well."

"Does your menstrual cycle make the headaches worse or better?"

"No, my cycle has no affect on whether or not I get a headache."

"Do you have any problem with urination or bowel movements?"

"No."

"Do you have any other problems or conditions other than the headaches?"

"No, Master Liu, nothing else, other than I am a little fat and I really would like to lose some weight. Do you think you can help me lose some weight?"

"It is possible, but losing weight requires a different approach. Yes, treatments and herbs will help you to balance your energy so your body will process food correctly. But it is also important to change your lifestyle, to eat the right foods at the appropriate time and to lead a balanced life that is consistent from day to day. Exercise is also important. Do you do Tai Chi Chuan or Qi Gong?"

"No, Master. I have no time to do it and, besides, there is no one competent enough to teach me."

"Tai Chi Chuan and Qi Gong have helped many people with muscular pain, headaches, depression, joint pain, and weight problems. You might want to consider it as a possible lifestyle change. Maybe I can find someone in the area to call on you to teach you Tai Chi Chuan. Would that be all right with you?"

"Yes, Master."

"Are you moody or do you feel your emotions are sometimes not right for the occasion?"

"No, I am not moody, but I often feel irritated, angry, and depressed. Many times, I do not know why I feel that way. My husband works very long hours. He is kind to me and the children. Many times this feeling comes on for no reason and is difficult to control. I do not even know how to explain it to my family. They may think I am making this all up or that it is all in my head. It is not enjoyable for them when I feel like this or have a bad headache. When it comes on, I just want to be left alone. It is better to lie down in a darkened room until it passes or I fall asleep."

"Can you point to the location in your head where you have the headaches?"

Liu looked at the spot where Mrs. Wang pointed and made a mental note of the location.

"The headache extends from the side close to the top of my head and down to the nape of my neck. The muscles on the side of my neck at the base of my skull really get sore. It is almost like the headache extends into the muscle."

"Pei Ke!"

"Yes, Master?"

"Are you paying attention?"

"Yes, Master."

"Mrs. Wang, would you please stick out your tongue."

Liu looked at Mrs. Wang's tongue. He considered the width of the tongue, the thickness of the tongue, the color of the tongue, the coating of the tongue, the color of both the tongue and its coating, and whether or not it had any distinguishing markings, such as grooves or indentations.

"Pei Ke, come look at her tongue. Notice that her tongue is a little redder than a normal tongue, and the coating of the tongue is slightly yellow."

Pei Ke looked and hoped he was noticing the right things.

"Mrs. Wang, I would like to feel your pulses," Liu said when Pei Ke had returned to his chair. She nodded.

Liu felt the pulses on both wrists for about one minute each.

"It appears you have a condition referred to as Liver Fire Rising. Pei Ke, I know this from the answers she gave me, my observation that she is a little flushed in the face, the look of her tongue, and the taut and rapid pulse." He turned back to Mrs. Wang.

"I don't know what that means," she said. "It sounds serious. Is there something wrong with my liver?"

"Do you drink much plum wine?"

"No, I don't drink any wine. But would you please talk to my husband and get him to stop drinking? Whenever his friends come late at night he stays up with them and they play Mah Jong until early morning. Then he opens the teahouse without getting any sleep. Many days it is all work and drinking. I get the feeling he does not even know I am here. I feel ignored."

Pei Ke could see the emotion in her face and could not decide if it was sadness, anger, or depression.

"I want to reassure you I don't think there is anything wrong with your liver," said Liu. "Your symptoms are quite common. This problem is more common in women than men and can be helped with either acupuncture or a combination of acupuncture and herbs. The liver energy in your body is rising upwards to your head, causing the headache. Since liver and gall bladder are coupled meridians, the Gall Bladder Meridian is also affected. The reason it is worse in the middle of the night is that the liver energy is at its maximum between one and three in the morning. After three in the morning, the liver energy starts to subside, thus the headache starts to subside."

"Are you sure there is nothing wrong with my liver or gall bladder?"

"They are both fine. It is just our way in medicine of identifying different patterns of energy excess or deficiency."

"Master, be truthful with me. How did I get this problem?"

"I cannot be sure unless I spent more time with you and watch your life style and eating habits. However, all of our health issues can be summarized into one word: imbalance. Correct the imbalance and your problem will be better. I am going to write a prescription for you to take to the herbalist. Acupuncture would also help. Would you like a treatment now?"

"Yes, please do what you think is best Master I just want the pain to go away and stay away. I will go to the temple and pray to Kuan Yin to bless you with good health."

Liu helped Mrs. Wang up from the chair and took her to the bed for her to lie down. He put a pillow under her head and raised her knees up with another pillow.

"Pei Ke, I want you to watch what I am doing. Because she has a condition of Liver Fire Rising, I am going to choose the following points. Xing Jian point is used because this point is one of the major points in relieving excess liver fire. Since this is an excess condition, characterized by a fullness and tightness in her liver pulse, it is appropriate to disperse the energy. The Liver Meridian runs from the large toe upwards to the body. This point is the second point on the Liver Meridian and is located on the top of the foot between the large toe and the next toe. It is about one half inch from the edge of the web between the toes. Now, from our previous discussion, which direction should I insert the needle?"

Pei Ke thought for a moment, trying to switch from listening to providing a response. He sensed that Mrs. Wang was watching and waiting for him to reply.

"Master, since the energy goes upward on the Liver Meridian and you want to decrease the energy, then the tip of the needle should be pointed towards the end of the toes."

"That is correct."

Out of the corner of his eye, Pei Ke could see a slight smile and a sense of relief on Mrs. Wang's face. He watched as Liu inserted the first needle in the acupuncture point on the right foot. He could see a slight muscle contraction in the area of the needle. He watched as the master put a needle in the same point on the opposite foot. In both cases, the needle was at an angle pointed towards the end of the big toe. Looking at Mrs. Wang, he could see no indication of pain, rather a slight sense of relief on her face.

"How do you feel now?" asked Liu.

"Oh, thank you. After you inserted the first needle, the pain diminished."

"Pei Ke, the next acupuncture point is Bai Hui. It is on the Governing Vessel Meridian. Since the meridian runs upward from the area of the anus, it is a single meridian. This point is located by extending an imaginary line from the bottom of the ear lobe to the top of the ear and then to the top of the head. Another imaginary line extends from the tip of the nose directly over the top of the head. Where these two imaginary lines intersect at the top of the head is where the acupuncture point is located. Do you remember me explaining how to locate this acupuncture point?"

"Yes, Master."

"I choose this point because the internal pathway of the energy of the Liver Meridian rises upward from the foot. It eventually gets to the eye by way of internal pathways. From the eye, it goes across the head to this point. Another reason for choosing this point is its calming effect on the mind."

Pei Ke watched as Liu inserted the needle into Mrs. Wang's scalp. He was sure she was going to feel this needle.

"How do you feel now," asked Liu.

"Is the needle in, Master?"

"Yes, the needle is in. How do you feel?"

"Master, you are so good at this, I didn't feel a thing and my head is feeling better. The sharpness of the headache is gone. The area of the headache is smaller and less intense."

"The next acupuncture point I am going to use is Tai Chong. It is the third acupuncture point of the Liver Meridian. It is located a little above the Xing Jian point close to where the two bones meet. I choose this point because it is classified as the source of the energy for this meridian, and I want to sedate this energy a little."

Pei Ke again watched as Liu carefully inserted needles on both of Mrs. Wang's feet. Liu continued the needling process choosing more points until he was finished.

"How do you feel now?"

Mrs. Wang shook her head and smiled. "The headache is gone. How long will it stay gone?"

"It depends on why it came in the first place. Your emotions play a significant factor in this type of headache. Try to be calm as much as possible and do not let things upset you. I'm going to write a prescription for some herbs for you to take for a few days. These herbs will continue the process started with the acupuncture. Now, is it all right for Pei Ke to ask some questions?"

"Yes."

"Pei Ke, what would you like to ask Mrs. Wang?"

"Mrs. Wang, I was watching you as Master Liu was inserting the needles. Was the treatment painful?"

"It was not painful at all. I knew that Master Liu was doing the acupuncture, but it was not uncomfortable."

"What did it feel like during the treatment?"

"Obviously, there was a sense of relief because the headache went away. It seemed like the headache melted away, followed by a sense of peacefulness. Another way of saying it is like something being drained from my head. You could also say there was an increased sense of well-being as the pain subsided." She turned to the master.

"Master Liu, is there another point or points you can use to make me feel more relaxed?"

"Yes, there are a number of points that can be chosen. Let me feel your pulse and see where the energy is now unbalanced."

Pei Ke watched as Liu felt the pulses on the radial artery of both wrists.

"Pei Ke, it is important for you to feel the pulses on her left wrist."

Pei Ke moved over to the left side of Mrs. Wang. Liu took Pei Ke's hand and gently placed his fingers on the appropriate places on the radial artery so Pei Ke could feel the pulses.

"Notice the differences in the pulses on the three pulse points?"

"Yes, Master. Some feel strong and some feel weak."

"The strong pulse is an indication of excess and the weak pulse is an indication of a deficiency. She still has an imbalance in her body."

Pei Ke watched as Liu continued the reading of the pulses. When he was done with the left side, he went to the right side and did the same thing.

He noticed Liu first placed the middle finger on the pulses followed by the index finger and then the ring finger. He moved the fingers so only one finger touched the radial artery at a time. In succession he went from the index finger to the middle finger and then to the ring finger. His first touch of each pulse point was light. Then he noticed Liu applying more pressure to the point and holding it for a period of time before relaxing the pressure. He did this a couple of times on each of the pulse points. Finally, he took two more needles and inserted them into a point on each wrist.

"How do you feel now?"

"A little more relaxed."

"Do you want to feel more relaxed?"

"Yes, please."

"How relaxed do you want to be?"

"I want to be as relaxed as possible. It was not enjoyable having this headache."

Liu touched the radial artery on each wrist one more time. He then began to touch an acupuncture point on the hand and foot. He did this with a combination of points, always touching both a leg and arm or a foot and hand. He would touch with only one finger and the touch seemed to be ever so light. Pei Ke could see the relaxation taking place in her body. Her shoulders dropped closer to the bed and whatever tension remained in the rest of her body seemed to melt away. It appeared she either had gone into a deep state of relaxation or had fallen asleep.

"How do you feel now?" asked Liu.

"I feel as if I am floating on this bed. I do not have a headache. It seems as if my body from neck down is completely gone. There is no feeling whatsoever."

"Is the feeling uncomfortable or does it make you feel uneasy in any way?"

"No, the feeling is like nothing I have experienced before. It is as if there is nothing. It can only be described as quite pleasurable. Maybe this is what the ancient Taoist monks referred to as nothingness." She touched his arm. "Master Liu, it is late; please stay with us for a few days."

"Thank you, but we need to leave in the morning. We have a long journey ahead of us and we must make as much progress as possible each day."

Because he was watching for it, Pei Ke noticed the master's hand drift to the message again and his face darken briefly. He did not think Mrs. Wang had noticed.

"Master Liu," she said, "as I mentioned before, our son has hurt his shoulder, and our daughter-in-law also gets headaches and has monthly abdominal pain."

"Yes, I will take care of both of them. For now, I want you to close your eyes and relax."

Pei Ke noted she was slurring her words as if she was going deeper into total muscle and mental relaxation.

Liu took Pei Ke over to the other side of the room where they could speak quietly and not disturb Mrs. Wang.

"Pei Ke, do you have any questions to ask while Mrs. Wang is relaxing?"

"Master, I have many questions, but I don't know where to begin. It all seems so unreal and mystical to me."

"There is nothing mystical about acupuncture. It does not violate any religious beliefs, morals, or philosophies, so it does not matter if you are Buddhist or Taoist or if you believe in any other philosophy or religion. It is only knowing, from many years of experience, what to do when the energy in the body is out of balance. Remember to balance the energy in the body. This allows the body to return to a natural condition based on that body's ancestral constitution.

"All of us in this profession started out the same way. Nobody is born an acupuncturist or doctor. It is only through diligent study and experience that we can help the patient."

Pei Ke nodded, then asked, "Master, what were you doing when you touched Mrs. Wang?"

"I was balancing the energy in her body through Qi Gong. I could also hold my hands over her body and derive somewhat the same effect. However, I wanted her to relax immediately, so I touched the points."

"Which points?"

"The ancients referred to these points as Turtle Points. You will learn them later. You need to know more about what these points are used for before you indiscriminately start touching the body. For example, I told you a little about the Xing Jian acupuncture point. Do you remember?"

"Yes, Master."

"As you saw I used the Tai Chong point also. This point is one of the Four Gate Points. It is the Yuan Point of the energy of the Liver Meridian."

"Master, do each of the points have so much to remember as the Tai Chong point?"

"All three hundred sixty-one points on the Classical Meridian system have a function. It is your responsibility to memorize this information as I give it to you, which is why I do not give it to you all at once. That is why I have a problem with those who are not fully trained in this art. They do not know the function of each one of the acupuncture points. For those not trained, it is just a selective approach that only works some of the time. They learn a little bit about this medicine and with good intentions want to use it. For example, it is widely known that the He Ku point on the hand in the web between the thumb and index finger is good for treating headaches, especially those headaches on the lateral side of the head; however, it is not always effective for all headaches.

"Your differential diagnosis must indicate whether this point should be used. If used inappropriately, the headache could become worse. Furthermore, this point is forbidden during certain stages of pregnancy because it can cause complications and fetal distress. The complications can become quite serious. The woman could lose her baby. Practitioners who lack adequate training do the patient a tremendous disservice."

Liu answered Pei Ke's questions for another fifteen minutes as Mrs. Wang rested peacefully.

"Mrs. Wang, it is time for you to get up. How do you feel now?"

Liu took out the needles and gave them to Pei Ke.

"I haven't felt this good in weeks, maybe even months. My headache is completely gone, and I feel as if I have had a good night's sleep."

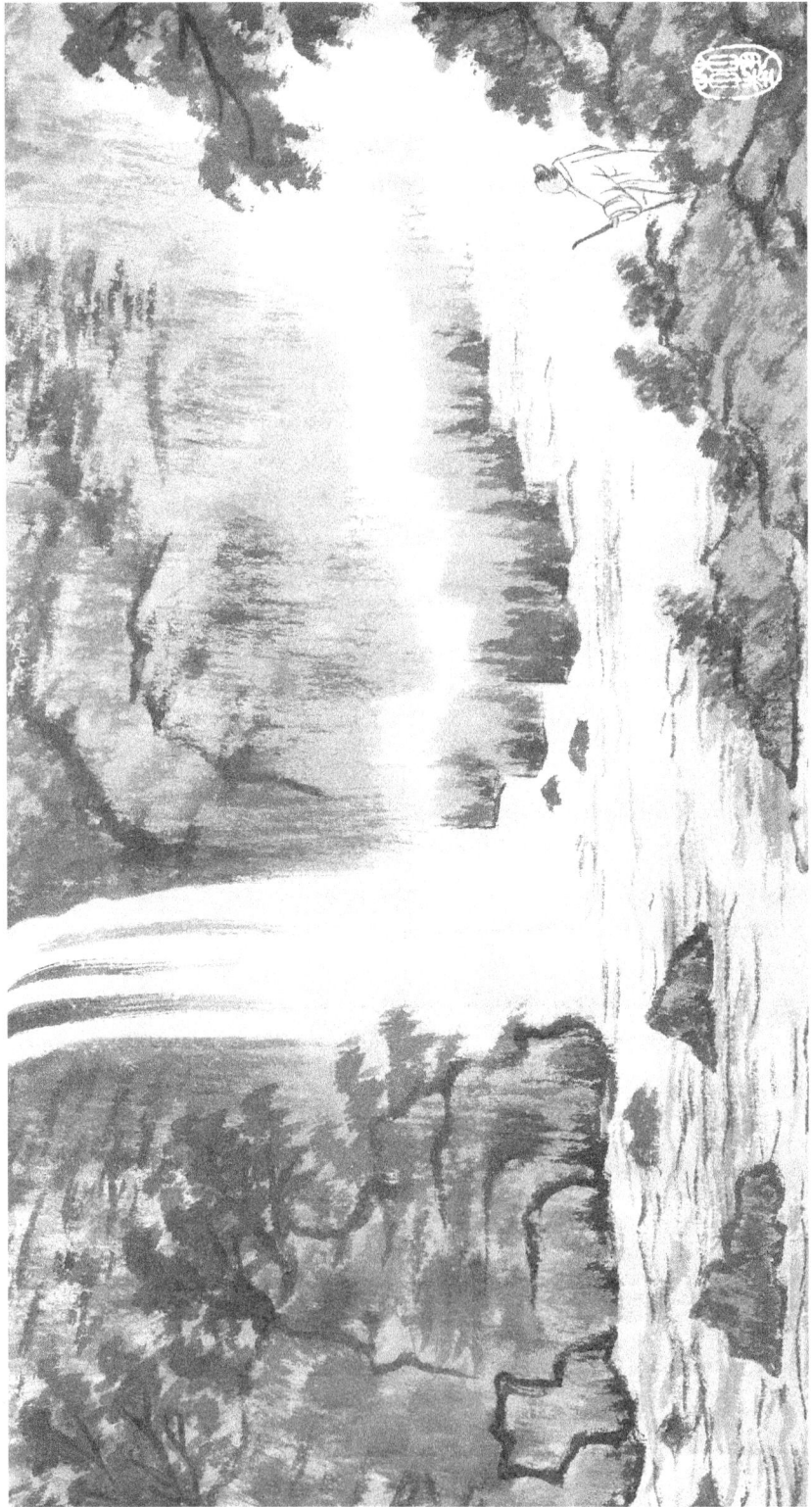

# CHAPTER SEVEN

Liu and Pei Ke left Mrs. Wang resting and walked slowly towards the son's quarters, stopping often to discuss acupuncture. It was the custom for the extended family to live under one roof, but in separate parts of the house. This was not true for the Wang family. When the teahouse was initially constructed, there was adequate room for the teahouse and living quarters for an extended family. As business improved, the teahouse expanded into the living quarters. Wang constructed separate but adjacent living quarters for the son and his family.

This arrangement was a blessing for the daughter-in-law who now had a little bit of privacy. It was customary for the daughter-in-law to wait on the mother–in-law for her every need. This relationship was abused by many mothers-in-law and thus caused ill feelings for a woman married into such a family. Quite often, conflict and anger existed between mother-in-law and the daughter-in-law. The separate building provided some distance between the families, allowing a measure of peace in the relationship.

The chilly night air invigorated the master and student as they walked in silence. Liu sensed an uneasiness about Pei Ke.

"You have any questions you want to ask about Mrs. Wang's treatment?" Liu asked. Pei Ke nodded.

"Keep the questions to what you saw tonight. It is fresh in your mind and you will want to reinforce what you have learned."

"Yes, Master. Is Mrs. Wang's problem common?"

"As I said, it is more common in women than men. Some men will have this problem, but because of the nature of a woman's energy, she is more often afflicted."

"Why is that?" asked Pei Ke.

"As I mentioned to you before, each meridian is associated with an emotion. The Liver Meridian is associated with anger and depression. In today's society, women have less opportunity to vent their emotions. Women feel they are in a vulnerable and somewhat helpless position. This feeling leads to anger and depression. If women, who suffered from this type of headache, could discuss their frustrations openly without fear of repercussions or reprisals they would probably have fewer headaches."

"In other words this is an emotional problem."

"I am not a hundred percent positive it is an emotional problem with her, but her emotions could be a contributing factor. As I told her, I would need to observe her more to be certain. If an emotional factor is involved, it could be related to her husband, the daughter-in-law, her son, or the responsibility and work she does around the home."

"So our emotions can affect our overall health?"

"Yes, definitely. More so than anyone would ever suspect. However, do not forget that other factors are just as important. For one person, an emotional factor could cause a headache. In another person, a similar emotional factor may not cause a headache. In a third person, something else could cause a headache. For Mrs. Wang, Liver Fire Rising caused the headache. If we delved a little deeper, the question would be what caused the Liver Fire Rising.

"Different symptoms indicate the diagnosis and treatment would be different. As an example, Mrs. Wang complained of insomnia, bitter taste in her mouth, throbbing headache, and pain in her eyes. If she had mentioned that her headache was more in the temples and that she had diarrhea, and her tongue was pale instead of red, the diagnosis would have been Liver Blood Deficiency.

"At first, this information does not seem to be important, but it is imperative to treat the problem correctly. Some of the acupuncture points used in treating Liver Fire Rising also treat Liver Blood Deficiency. In addition, I would use other acupuncture points to treat that problem. The herbal formula for treating Liver Fire Rising is different than the formula for treating Liver Blood Deficiency."

"Master, do you mean the signs and symptoms of a disease can be the same except for one or two determining factors?"

"Exactly. That is why an inadequately trained doctor assumes all headaches can be treated the same way with the same points and medications. This type of doctor is doing the patient a tremendous disservice."

"How does one remember all that information and get it correct each time?"

"It is like anything else we do. How does the sculptor or artist know which techniques are the right techniques? It is only through correct practice that this art is mastered. I know you think it is an impossible chore, but think what you now know about Liver Fire Rising, and how to distinguish this ailment from Liver Blood Deficiency."

As they walked, Pei Ke considered his master's encouragement. It was true, he now knew about Liver Fire Rising and how it affects women. He also knew the distinguishing factors to isolate Liver Blood Deficiency. Of course, if all these factors are important, there must be hundreds of determining factors one must memorize in order to do the patient no harm.

"Master, what would happen if someone treated the patient for the wrong thing? For example, what if we had treated Mrs. Wang for Liver Blood Deficiency rather than Liver Fire Rising?"

"In that case, using acupuncture points for Liver Blood Deficiency instead of acupuncture points for Liver Fire Rising would only give Mrs. Wang minimal relief, rather than the total relief she experienced. She would feel some relief, of course, because some of the points are common to both conditions, but there are separate points for each condition as well. The same applies to herbal formulas."

"How often should Mrs. Wang have treatments?"

"A series of treatments would help her even more but we must leave in the morning. The acupuncture has helped to correct the imbalance in her body. The herbal formula will go further in enhancing the Qi so the problem will be less severe. If we could stay, I would do more treatments on her."

"Will Mrs. Wang's problem completely disappear?"

"It is a difficult question for me to answer. Since there is an underlying emotional problem, it depends on how her constitution reacts to the treatment. It would help if she could get to the source of the problem."

"Does she know the source?"

"Maybe not, but I will tell her before we leave what I feel she needs to do to solve this problem. She may not take my suggestions but at least she will know what is happening. Often, just being aware of the problem keeps the problem from manifesting itself as a pain symptom."

―――――――

Pei Ke and Liu continued walking across the courtyard. As they approached the residence, Wang Shen Men, Wang's son met them at the door.

"Master Liu, it is an honor for you to visit with us. Please come in."

"It is very kind of your father to give us a place to stay for the evening." He introduced Pei Ke and the two young men exchanged pleasantries.

"We were visiting with your mother and she said that you and your wife had some health issues. Since we are staying here, maybe I can help."

"Master, my problem is nothing of major concern. I have some minor shoulder pain from a fall which took place a couple of months ago. It is my wife who needs your help. Please come in and make yourself comfortable. I will go get her. She is not feeling well and is resting in bed."

The son's residence was not as elaborate as the parents'. Even so, their quarters were opulent compared to almost all but the wealthy. The son's comfortable home was yet another example of how well Wang was doing as owner of the teahouse. Various scrolls of calligraphy decorated the walls. Some were quite good while others were only there to remind the son and daughter-in-law of their duty to the family. Reminders in Chinese culture of the Confucian philosophy of right and wrong and the duty one has to honor their ancestors were everywhere. Liu liked what he saw in this home.

As Liu and Pei Ke were looking at the various scrolls, Wang's son returned. "Master, my wife says her pain is quite bad. Would you mind coming to the bedroom to see her?"

"Of course," Liu said.

As the three of them walked down the hallway, Pei Ke again marveled at the richness of the quarters. He hoped some day he might be as wealthy as this. He was a good person. He paid respect to the ancestors. Why did some have money and wealth and others have virtually nothing? It was not fair. Of course, there were those like Liu who did not want anything. They seemed to be happy in their poverty. Maybe Liu was happy he had nothing. Then he did not have to worry about someone trying to steal his wealth. He seemed to know wealthy people, and his family must be wealthy, but he eschewed the wealth for himself. Of course, he knew his brother would give him some money if he asked. If they had wealth they must have land, and lots of it.

As they entered the bedroom, Wang introduced his wife Sha Mei to Liu and Pei Ke. She lay beneath some blankets. Liu immediately knew she was not feeling well. She looked as if she meant to be happy but the effort was more than she could make.

Liu motioned for Pei Ke to stay at the foot of the bed as he walked over to the side of the bed.

"We have come from your mother-in-law's quarters. She was not feeling well but is resting now," said Liu.

"What is the matter with her?" Sha Mei asked.

"We all have our health issues. It is best you ask her for yourself," Liu said. "She told us that you have complained of headaches."

"Yes, I have headaches every once in a while. It is not the headaches that bother me, though. It is the time of the month that bothers me."

"What are your symptoms?"

Sha Mei first looked at Pei Ke, then at Liu, and finally at her husband. Instinctively, she pulled the covers closer to her chin.

"Pei Ke is my student. He is learning how to be a doctor. You can trust him to be professional. If you approve, I would like him to assist me in your treatment."

She nodded slowly.

"I have painful menstrual cramps every month. The cramps are so bad I have to lie down."

"How long have you been having these cramps?"

"For many years. They are getting worse as I get older. I know I sound like an old lady."

"Sha Mei, I need to ask you some very personal questions so I can determine the nature of this problem. Please do not be embarrassed by my questions."

She smiled weakly.

"Master Liu, I am already embarrassed having you and your student here in my bedroom."

"Your husband is here with us, so there is no problem."

"Master Liu, it is not you, it is just the idea of sharing my most personal information with someone else."

"I understand," said Liu. "How old are you?"

"I am twenty-one."

" How old were you when you first started menstruating?"

"I was eleven."

"When did you first start having severe cramping?"

"When I was thirteen. Actually, I was uncomfortable right from the start, but the cramping has worsened over the years. Can you help me?"

"Yes, I think I can help as long as I have enough information to make a decision."

"I don't want to continue like this. It is very painful for the first two days. No one understands how bad it feels unless they have had this same problem. I complain to my mother-in-law about the headaches, but it is not just headaches, it is the cramps that really bother me. Everyone wants to be sympathetic, but there is nothing they can do. They probably feel as helpless as I do."

"How many days does your period last?

"About five or six days."

"Do you have cramping only at the beginning or throughout the whole time?"

"Only for the first couple of days."

"Do you have any breast tenderness?"

"Yes, some, but I could tolerate that if the cramping would just go away."

"What color is the menses?"

"It is a normal red color, but there are large clots at the beginning."

"Does it feel better if you put a warm towel on your abdomen?"

"Yes. How did you know that?"

"There are many signs and symptoms which help me to narrow the problem to a specific condition. I am trying to isolate the cause now. Do you have any special tastes in your mouth during this time of the month?"

"No, but I really crave sweet things just before the period starts and for the first day or so. I can always tell by the cravings that my period is going to start. It is almost uncontrollable. I have to force myself not to eat those things. I know too much sweet is not good for me."

"You are right. Too much of anything is not good for you. Everything must be in balance. In Chinese medicine, the spleen is associated with blood and therefore deals with menstruation. Sugar or sweet things are related with spleen. When the cycle is ready to start, the spleen becomes active and there is a craving."

"Does this craving happen to just me or does it happen to all women?"

"It doesn't happen to all women, but it does happen to many. As you know, the female body goes through many changes during its cycle, and those changes are more difficult for some women."

"What is causing my problem?"

"I am trying to find out now. Do you feel hot during menstruation?"

"No, not especially, but it feels good to lie down. The discomfort is not quite so bad then."

"Do you have any pain in your lower back at this time?"

"Yes."

"Is it sore now?"

"Yes." Sha Mei removed the covers and pointed to the area of her back that was sore, just along her waistline.

"That area of your back is where the kidneys are located. The spleen is not the only organ affected by your monthly period, but also the kidneys and liver. The ancient texts mention that the spleen controls the blood, the liver stores the blood, and the kidney governs reproduction. These three meridians are all Yin in nature and are located on the inside of your leg leading upwards into your abdominal area."

"So do I have a problem with my spleen, liver, or kidneys?"

"Not necessarily. Let me ask you some more questions. What color is your urine?"

"Why is that important?" She blushed.

"If the color of the urine is pale, it means one thing and if it is dark, it means another. It would change during the course of the energy imbalance causing your problem. All these questions when taken together mean something. It is not appropriate to isolate each symptom to arrive at a diagnosis. It is only the sum of all the symptoms that leads us to the right conclusion. I know my questions may seem meaningless, but when you understand that each symptom is due to an energy imbalance, you will appreciate my detailed questions. Changing two of the symptoms could alter my diagnosis, and therefore the treatment pattern."

"My urine is pale in color."

"Do you have any strange smells?"

"No. But food is the last thing I want while in bed."

"Can you point to the area where the discomfort is greatest?"

Pei Ke watched as Sha Mei pointed to the area on her abdomen. Liu carefully touched the spot and pushed down on the area.

"Does my pushing in this area make it feel worse or better?"

"Neither. It feels the same."

"Please stick out your tongue. Pei Ke, come look at her tongue. It is a classic tongue for this type of condition."

Pei Ke took a couple of steps to the side of the bed and looked at Sha Mei's tongue. He noticed the coating on the tongue was slightly different than the coating on Mrs. Wang's tongue.

"Pei Ke, what do you notice about Sha Mei's tongue?"

"The tongue itself is slightly pale and the coating on the tongue is white."

"You are correct. What else?"

"There are no grooves on the side of the tongue."

"If there were grooves what would that indicate?"

"It would mean a possible phlegm problem."

"Very good."

"Sha Mei, I am going to feel your pulses to see if there are any energy imbalances."

Pei Ke watched as Liu first felt the pulses on the woman's right wrist. He placed his middle finger on the pulse with a light touch on the superficial pulse followed by a more forceful touch on the deep pulse. Liu then went to the other two pulses, taking a minute or two with each to get an accurate reading. He next went to the left.

"Sha Mei, I know you are most concerned with the cramps, but tell me more about the headaches associated with your cycle. Do you get headaches at any other time?"

"I will occasionally have a headache, but it is rare and does not concern me. I understand everyone gets an occasional headache."

"Where are the headaches?"

"They are located on the sides of my head."

"Is the pain dull or throbbing?"

"My headache throbs on both sides at the same time, but only for the first part of my cycle. It almost always goes away once the menses starts."

"When you are lying in bed, is there any position which is more comfortable for your back?"

"Each time it is different. Sometimes it is best to lie on my back in a darkened room and wait for the headache to go away. Other times there is no comfortable position."

"When you are not having your period, do you have any unusual vaginal discharge?"

"No, once the period is over I am all right, though I know some women have constant discharge."

Liu nodded.

"There are specific reasons for constant vaginal discharge. The problem is treatable with acupuncture and herbal formulations."

She glanced at her husband then said, "We want to have children, but I have not been able to conceive. Do you think that is part of my problem?"

"Your problem is multi-faceted. I will try to take care of you, but to answer your question, all health issues can be simplified to an imbalance of the Yin and Yang. If we can correct the imbalance, your health issues will go away, including your inability to conceive."

Sha Mei fell quiet for a moment, but Pei Ke could tell she wanted to speak. He suspected a similar expression had crossed his face many times before.

"Is there something else?" Master Liu said, perceptive as always.

"Yes, Master Liu. Having you here and listening to you talk of Chinese medicine reminds me of some issues that I heard of from friends and family. Do you mind if I ask you about them?"

"I do not mind. You may ask me anything."

"Thank you." She bowed slightly, even though she was lying down. "My mother had eight children. Now she cannot control her urine. When she coughs, sneezes, or laughs, she leaks a little. She has to wear pads, which she changes quite often. Is there something you could do to help her?"

"Yes. She has what is called incontinence, a common problem for women who have had multiple children. The bladder falls due to a Qi deficiency. The Qi is not rising on the Conception Vessel Meridian, and therefore the area of the bladder is deficient. Acupuncture and Chinese herbs are very effective in treating this problem. Does she live close by?"

"No. She lives a few miles from here. I only see her every other month."

"Tell her to see an acupuncturist. He will be able to take care of this problem."

"I'm glad to hear it. I also have a close friend that I see quite often. She has just had her third child but she does not produce enough milk for the baby. Is there anything she can do for this problem?"

"Yes. This problem can be solved with diet, acupuncture and herbs."

"Do you have to put needles into her breasts?"

"I could not say for sure until I had done a differential diagnosis, but this problem is most likely another Qi problem. An acupuncturist will probably put some needles in the center of her chest, under her breasts, on the side of her breast, in her little finger, and on her legs."

"Do you put one in the nipple?"

"No, there is an acupuncture point on the nipple, but it is forbidden to be needled. It is more of a landmark point for locating some other points. There are several forbidden points on the body. They are usually forbidden for certain types of conditions. As an example, if a patient has a fever then heat therapy is not used. If the patient has hypertension some points cannot be used. A well-trained acupuncturist knows all of this."

"Master Liu, another friend had terrible morning sickness when she was pregnant. It lasted for about three months. She was sick all day long. Can that be treated?"

"Yes. That can be treated successfully with acupuncture and herbs. Pregnancy should be a time of joy and happiness and not a time of sickness. Again it is an imbalance of Yin and Yang that needs correcting."

Pei Ke spoke before thinking, his fascination with his master's words spilling out in his words.

"Master, where are the acupuncture points for treating morning sickness?"

Liu looked reprovingly at his student, but he noticed that Sha Mei was nodding her head in interest as well, so he answered.

"Each situation is different, but in general the points are located on the arms and legs. During pregnancy, acupuncture should not be done on the woman's abdomen, as these points are forbidden during this time. In addition, some acupuncture points are contraindicated during pregnancy. However, acupuncture is safe during pregnancy for both the woman and her unborn child. Just make sure the acupuncturist is well trained in the specific technique of treating morning sickness. Now, are there any more questions?" He glanced at his student to suggest that this was not a general invitation.

"Yes, Master," Sha Mei said. "I am sorry for asking so many questions but I have never had the opportunity to ask. Another friend has been married for three years and she has not had any children. Can acupuncture help with that problem?"

"Yes, a combination of acupuncture and herbal formulas is very effective in treating infertility. Many women have fertility problems. Typically, it is again an energy imbalance on the Spleen Meridian, Kidney Meridian, and Liver Meridian. Once the energy is balanced, her body will be more viable for conception to take place. I have treated numerous women for this problem and have been quite successful. Sometimes it is not a problem with the woman, but a problem with the husband. There are acupuncture points and herbs to promote the male essence."

"Master, just one more question. I just thought of a friend who is pregnant and has developed lower back pain. The pain is quite severe and extends from her back down the side of her leg."

"It is most likely sciatic nerve pain. It is easily treated with acupuncture. Your friend does not need to suffer during her pregnancy."

Pei Ke listened as Liu continued to ask Sha Mei a series of additional questions. His questioning became very detailed and specific, almost as if he were trying to differentiate between two different possibilities. After asking all his questions, he started inserting needles into Sha Mei. Right from the beginning with the first few needles, her face changed as the pain started to melt away. Her body relaxed and her shoulders, which were tense, relaxed into the bed. Her legs, originally drawn up became relaxed.

Tears came to her eyes as the pain departed from her abdomen and lower back. Pei Ke wondered how terrible the pain must have been. He surmised she had not slept well for several days. How difficult to go through that pain each month. Pei Ke was thankful he was a man, but he wanted to be able to help someone like her. He remembered his mother who had similar problems.

"Master, it is true what my mother said about you!" remarked Wang's son. "She said you work miracles, and I have just seen my first miracle. Thank you for taking care of my wife. We are indebted to you forever."

"I am happy to be able to do this for you and your wife."

"Will she need more treatments?"

"Yes. Usually with this kind of abdominal pain during her menses, she will need about three more treatments. Start the treatments just before her period. I will also write an herbal prescription for her to take now, and again each month for the next three months. Hopefully, this will help solve the problem."

"I will take the prescription to the herbalist in the morning."

"I would like her to rest now." Liu turned to Wang's son. "Is there somewhere we can go so she can rest in peace?"

"Yes, follow me."

Wang first walked to the side of the bed and touched his wife on the forehead. She opened her eyes and smiled. Pei Ke could tell there was a deep love between them. Wang Shen Men motioned for Liu and Pei Ke to follow him as he turned to leave the room. He looked back once and smiled as he saw the peacefulness in his wife. Then they went to the sitting area and Wang Shen Men motioned for them to sit.

"Your mother told me you are having some shoulder problems. Maybe I can help," said Liu.

"Master, you have done enough for one night. I am forever grateful that you have helped Sha Mei."

"Let me see what I can do. Where is the pain?"

"It is in my left shoulder. It hurts all the time, but hurts more when I raise my arm. The higher I lift my arm, the more intense the pain. It is almost impossible to raise my hand above my shoulder. It seems to catch or freeze up when I try."

"How did you hurt your shoulder?"

"I was working in the teahouse and I needed to lift some benches. They were just too heavy for me. As I was lifting one of them, it slipped from my grasp and hit my shoulder as I fell."

"How long have you had this pain?"

"For a couple of months. At first, it started to get better, but now from constant use it is just as bad as before. When I just let my arms relax on the table it hurts less, at least."

"Have you ever had a neck injury?"

"No. What does my neck have to do with my shoulder?"

"I have found when someone has pain in their wrist, forearm, elbow, or shoulder; quite often it is due to a neck injury. In the process of treating the neck, the pain in the arm, shoulder, and wrist will go away. This is especially true when there is pain in the forearm and wrist from repetitive finger, wrist, or hand motion. Sometimes it is nothing more than a tight muscle in the upper back, which has gone into spasm from overuse. Do you have any other pains?"

"No, the problem is just in my left shoulder."

Pei Ke listened as Liu went through a series of questions similar to the questioning he had done with Mrs. Wang and her daughter-in-law. After questioning, he moved Wang Shen Men's arm and listened for any sounds. He felt the area for heat. Next he felt the area to see if there was a popping sensation.

"Does it hurt in your right hip?"

"No, Master."

Liu again felt in the shoulder area as he moved the left arm one direction, than another.

"When you move my arm, the pain is right there," said Wang Shen Men as he pointed to a spot on his shoulder.

"Pei Ke, pay close attention to what I do."

Liu felt Wang Shen Men's right hip and pressed firmly against the skin with the knuckle of his index finger.

"Master, that point is really sore. How did you know it was sore?"

Liu stepped back so he could look directly at Wang Shen Men.

"I remember what my first acupuncture teacher told me many years ago. He said, 'if there is a pain on the top, you need to treat on the bottom. If there is pain on the bottom, you need to treat on the top. If there is a pain on the left, you need to treat on the right. If there is pain on the right, you need to treat on the left. If there is pain on the front, you need to treat on the back; and if there is pain on the back you need to treat on the front.' It sounds very simple but it is rather profound. Pei Ke, here is a fast way to remember the protocol. If there is pain on the patient's right thumb, the treatment point is going to be on the patient's left big toe. If there is pain on the patient's right wrist, the treatment points are on the patient's left ankle. Based on what I just told you, if a patient has pain on their right knee where would you look for the treatment point?"

Pei Ke thought for a moment. "On the patient's left elbow?"

"If the pain is on the inside of the right knee where would you look for the pain on the patient's elbow? Would it be on the inside of the elbow or on the outside of the elbow?"

"It would be on the inside of the patient's left elbow," said Pei Ke.

"That is correct. This logic will help you solve many pain problems. It is not the only protocol, but it does help. It is also necessary to balance the energy in the patient's body to get the maximum result."

"Does this mean if someone has a headache, you can treat the feet and it will help the headache?"

"Yes, that is true. In fact one of the major acupuncture points for treating hemorrhoids is on top of the head."

"Does that mean if someone has a headache, the acupuncture point is located near the rectum?"

"Yes, it is possible to use a point near the rectum to treat certain types of headaches, but for modesty reasons there are better points."

Pei Ke thought for a moment of different possibilities. He smiled at some of the weird possibilities, but thought better of asking Liu.

"Is there pain here in your right leg just below the knee?" asked Liu as he pushed on an acupuncture point on Wang Shen Mei's leg.

"Yes, that point is sore. How did you know that?" asked Wang Shen Men.

"That point is on the Stomach Meridian, but it is associated with the internal pathway of the Large Intestine Meridian. Since the Large Intestine Meridian runs in close proximity to where the pain is in your shoulder, this point can be sore. It is found on the opposite side of the body."

"Can you fix my shoulder pain?" Wang asked.

"Yes, I think so, but I need to ask you some more questions."

Pei Ke listened as Liu continued to probe. Once he was satisfied about the answers, he had Wang lie down and inserted needles into Wang's hip, shoulder, and leg.

"You will need to lie here for about fifteen to twenty minutes. Just rest now."

Liu took hold of Pei Ke's arm and guided him away from Wang Shen Men. "Do you have any questions?"

"Yes, Master, though I think I understood everything you said. It is interesting how pain has many different facets. So far tonight we have treated three different kinds of pain. In the case of the shoulder pain, would it be possible to treat the pain with acupressure instead of acupuncture?"

"Yes, it would be possible. Acupressure would be appropriate for those instances where the injury is not structural and has not endured for very long. The longer the pain has lasted, the more difficult it is to treat with acupressure."

"Master, this information about how to locate points is very valuable, especially for martial arts practitioners."

"Yes, however acupressure can be used for many types of pain. It would not be good for Mrs. Wang's pain, nor would it be appropriate for the pain Sha Mai has. Both of their pain is more internal. Wang Shen Men's pain is more muscular. Now, here is another way to understand this technique of opposites. Visualize the patient standing with his feet apart and his arms above his head, like he was making an 'X'. Wherever you have the pain draw a line from the pain location through the belly button to the opposite side of the body. Do you understand?"

"Yes, Master. That is an easier way to think about it. Does this always work?"

"No, but it works enough that you will have success in treating many different types of pain problems."

"Master, it seems that women have more problems than men."

"The nature of women is different from the nature of men. They have unique energy patterns that we do not have. These energy patterns can often become unbalanced."

"Why?"

"They can become unbalanced due to lifestyle."

"Can you give me an example of an unbalanced lifestyle that would affect a woman and cause her to have these types of problems?"

"A good example would be drinking too many cold drinks, especially around the time when her period starts. The coldness depletes the Qi in the body. When it is winter time, do your muscles work well, or do they work better in the summer time?"

"In the winter my muscles are stiff because of the cold."

"The same thing applies to a woman's abdomen. When she drinks cold things, the body does not work correctly. The body needs warmth to function correctly. Also eating the wrong foods consistently will affect the woman. Some foods are cold in nature, and there are some foods that are warm in nature. Eating too much of the cold-type of foods causes the menstruation process to be affected. Lack of exercise and inadequate sleep will also affect a woman adversely. Stress and emotional factors also have an effect."

"We men don't have as many problems that women have," said Pei Ke.

"Yes, that is true, but men do have problems. The most significant problem men have is kidney deficiency. The kidney deficiency can come about through too much sexual activity, especially with different partners. The ancient Taoists believed each man had a set number of orgasms. This number diminished as the man grew older. The ancients believed each ejaculation would drain away some kidney energy. If a man had too many orgasms, especially at an early age, he would drain too much kidney energy. Once all the kidney energy is drained, the man would probably die. Kidney energy is associated with the lower back. Those who have continual lower back pain might think about curtailing their bedroom activities."

"Do women have a loss of kidney energy?"

"Yes, women have a loss of kidney energy, but not through orgasm as men do. They lose kidney energy through childbirth. Thus, bearing too many children would be detrimental to a woman. Some think too few children could also be detrimental; however, I have not seen that to be true."

"So if a man never has sex, he should be quite healthy and should live to an old age, right?"

"Yes, in theory, but it is not the way the male body was designed. The male body was designed to be part of the reproductive process. If there is a curtailment of bedroom activities, then there is a buildup of sexual energy. Qi Gong, Taoist Meditation, and Buddhist Meditation are helpful in regulating that build up. Abstinence is okay as long as you know what to do to regulate the buildup of the excess energy."

"Is this part of your secret to a healthy life?"

"Yes, it is part of the secret, but there are other aspects I will share with you as you develop your internal Qi. Developing this internal Qi is a process you have to go through. It is not possible to jump to the end of the process without experiencing the beginning and intermediate steps."

"So should I stay single or should I get married and have children?"

"Only you can answer that question. The training you are receiving now will be beneficial regardless of what you do. Just remember if you do get married, do nothing to excess."

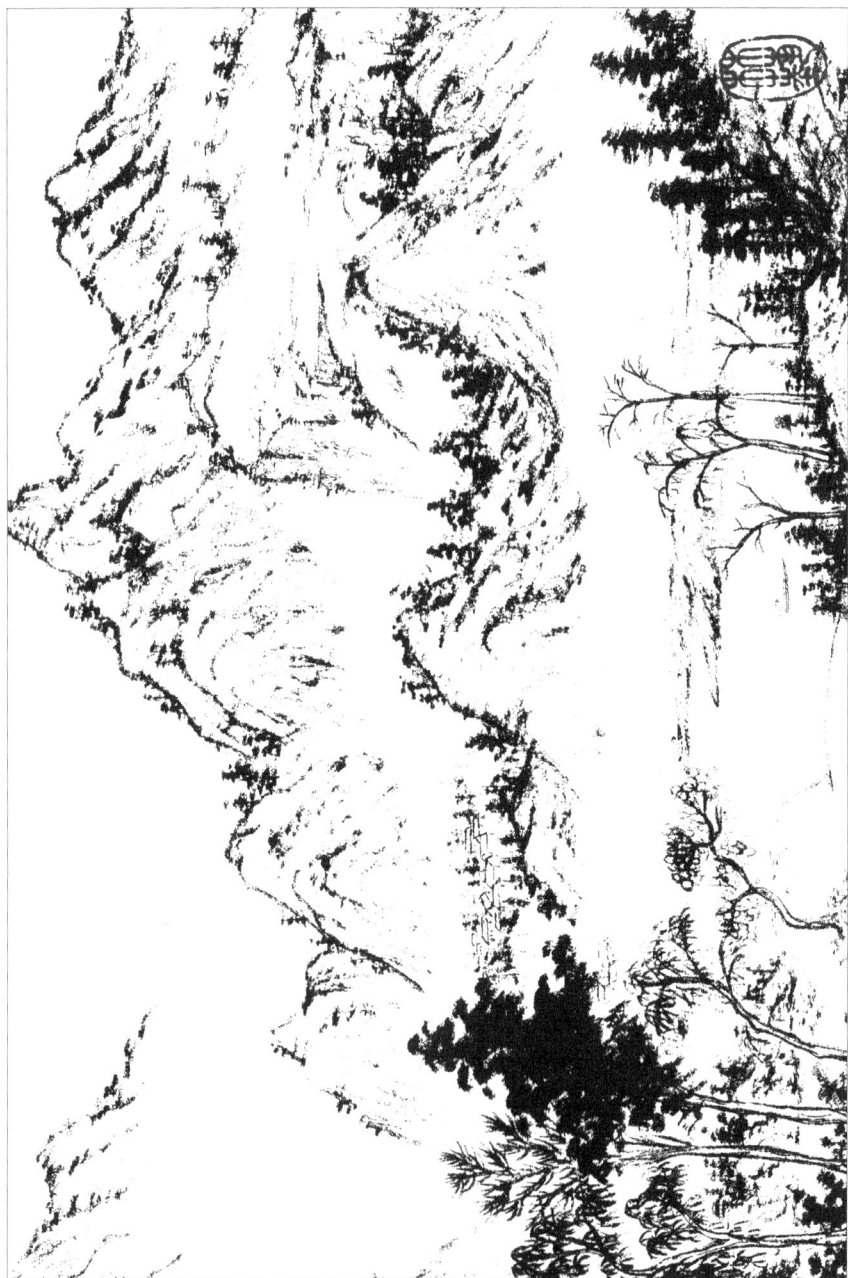

# CHAPTER EIGHT

After Liu and Pei Ke finished with Wang Shen Men and his wife, they walked back to Mrs. Wang's quarters. Pei Ke noted the wind blew from the south but it was still cool. When they arrived at Mrs. Wang's quarters, Liu tapped lightly on the door but there was no response.

"I suspect she has gone to bed and is in a deep sleep," said Liu. "She will sleep very well tonight, as will the other two. Tomorrow they will rise feeling much better and maybe a little different."

"Why will they feel better?" asked Pei Ke. "I mean, I know they had treatments, but does acupuncture work that fast?"

"It depends on many factors: the diagnosis, the length of the time they have had the problem, how they respond to treatments, the expertise of the doctor, and how well the treatment was administered. In general, the longer someone has a problem, the more difficult it is to solve. This is why one should think of these treatments as therapy rather than a onetime cure-all visit. Granted some patients are completely cured after one treatment, but that does not happen all the time."

Liu and Pei Ke returned to the teahouse. The full moon was visible, and the wind shifted to the north, making the walk chillier than before.

"I must further answer your question about why they will feel different for you to fully understand what has taken place," Liu said as they walked through the compound. "All that acupuncture can do is to start a healing process in the body. I hope that the healing process has begun for these people. The body, in theory, has the capacity to heal itself if given the chance. Treatment unblocks a flow of energy that has been blocked. Think of the acupuncturist as a facilitator in this whole process. I facilitate the healing of the body. It can then do what nature intended for the body to do. That is, to heal itself. Do you understand?"

Pei Ke thought for a moment before speaking. He tried to absorb all Liu had said. "If I understand you correctly, you have not healed anything but only started a process of healing."

"That is one way of looking at it. However, your patients will not think about it that way. They want to think you are the doctor and the healer, which you are. The term doctor is equated with healing. However, many so called doctors do not heal. They cover up the problem or suppress the symptoms. Then the problem is only alleviated for a short period until it comes back. Or, it does not go away at all. Some doctors only practice for the money. There is nothing wrong with earning a living from this practice, as long as you are competent in what you are doing."

"Master, you do not charge anything."

"I am not concerned with the money. Money is the root of much disharmony, which is the opposite of what I personally want to accomplish in life. If I acquire many things in life then I have to spend a certain amount of time worrying about what will happen with these things. I have to keep track of these things and worry about someone stealing them. If I have nothing, I do not have to be concerned. Instead I want to be free to meditate and study. Cultivating internal energy and having freedom to come and go as I please are very important to me. I understand this goes against the philosophy of most people, but I chose this way long ago and it has kept me happy, young, and productive. But everything has to be in balance. If everyone wanted to be an owner of a teahouse, there would be too many teahouses and no patrons to support the teahouse. If everyone wanted to be a monk, there would be too many monks. Someday you will have to make a choice."

"I do not want to be poor," Pei Ke said to himself. "That is my choice in life."

———————

Mr. Wang was not in the teahouse when Liu and Pei Ke entered. The girls were expecting them, however, and showed the two travelers to the guest quarters.

The guest quarters, which resembled a study area for students, were elaborately furnished, almost to the point of being ostentatious. The large open room had two beds in one corner concealed by two highly ornate and richly decorated screens. Liu recognized the carvings on the screens were depicting the Eight Taoist Immortals of antiquity.

In the center of the room, a table faced the entrance. On the table were calligraphy and painting brushes, along with different types of rice paper. An ink stone and ink stick lay on the table close to the rice paper. Pei Ke sensed both had been used recently. Artwork filled the room. Liu saw paintings from very famous ancient painters and calligraphers. If these scrolls were the originals, they were very valuable. Exquisite vases of all sizes sat on the floor or on luxuriously designed furniture. Carvings of ivory and jade added to the feeling of wealth. All the furniture and adornments followed the concepts of Feng Shui except that there was too much of everything. Wang must be cautious about who he allowed to use this room. Whoever entered would have to be a trusted friend. The temptation to steal something would be too great for just anyone.

Pei Ke had never seen so much artwork in one room. He thought the teahouse business must be a good business. Maybe he should apprentice himself to Wang. On second thought, Wang's son would inherit this business. Maybe he could learn from Wang and then set up his own business in another city.

"Pei Ke," said Liu. "I want you to look at this scroll."

Pei Ke walked from where he was standing to where Liu was looking intently at a multi-colored painting.

"The painting is beautiful," said Pei Ke. "I wish I could paint like that."

"This painting is unique. Do you see the message in the painting?"

Pei Ke looked at the scroll. On close examination, he could see the exquisite detail the artist put into the landscape. The placement of the trees, animals, and people blended into one harmonious and idealistic setting.

"This painting probably summarizes Wang's true desire," Liu said. "Either a close friend gave him this piece or someone painted it for him."

He moved slightly away from the painting so Pei Ke could examine it.

"There are five blessings in Chinese culture, Pei Ke. They are good fortune, prosperity, longevity, happiness, and good health. Of these five, good fortune and longevity are considered the most important and of these, longevity is regarded as the highest. This painting is unusual because its theme is entirely depicting the concept of longevity."

Liu moved back to Pei Ke. The young man still studied the picture.

"What do you see as the most prominent feature of the painting?" asked Liu.

"The painting has a physical depth to it."

"Note the turtle," said Liu. "The ancients believed the turtle lived to be about one thousand years old. Thus, the placement of the turtle in the painting blesses the recipient to live a long life. Pine trees live to be very old. China has virgin forests where the trees are so wide at the base that it takes many men to put their arms around the tree. Therefore, in this painting the pine trees also indicate longevity. If you look closely, you can see that one of the children is holding a piece of fruit. Usually, the fruit is a peach, which is another symbol of longevity. The rocks in the foreground last forever and indicate blessing for longevity to the recipient of the painting. A crane flies overhead. Cranes mate for life and live for many years. The God of Longevity is riding on a crane—another symbol of longevity. The butterflies indicate longevity as do the Eight Taoist Immortals off to one side." He paused, allowing Pei Ke to take in the symbolism, then asked, "Now that you see the longevity aspects of the painting, what is your impression of the work?"

"Knowing something about the meaning of the painting enhances its beauty."

"Yes, it is nice. However, you should also note that in this case, the concept of longevity is excessive. From a Taoist point of view, the Yin and Yang should always be in balance. This painting depicts the extreme. When Yin or Yang extend to their extremes, they change in nature to the opposite. Thus Yin to its extreme will change into Yang, and Yang to its extreme will change into Yin."

Liu stepped over to the next painting and looked at it for a few moments before speaking.

"Do you see the two men playing a board game here?"

Not another painting, thought Pei Ke. He had been walking all day, and was tired, and Master wanted to give him a painting lesson. Didn't *he* ever get tired?

"Yes, they are playing on a block of wood," Pei Ke said. "I have seen men in the park playing the game for hours, but I have never played it. Have you?"

"It is a fascinating game. It is played on a grid of sixteen squares by sixteen squares. You place black or white pebbles on the grid at the intersection of the lines. The object of the game is to surround your opponent's pebbles with your pebbles."

"Master, it looks as if two games are being played. Two other men in the painting are also playing the same game. Do you see them?"

"Yes, the scroll depicts two sets of games. However, the second game is a little different. You can tell by the layout of the stones. The second game is played on the same board, but the object of the game is much different and much simpler. To win, all you need to do is get five stones in a row—either horizontally, vertically, or diagonally."

"Master, all you need to win is to place five stones in a row?"

Pei Ke turned away from the painting to face Liu. He saw a faint smile on Liu's face.

"Yes, that is correct. We would take turns playing a stone. Either white or black would start first. Each time you had two or more stones in a row I would put a stone to block the row so you could not get more than five stones in a row."

"That does not seem difficult."

"Yes, the game seems very simple, but requires you to be able to look or think ahead two to three moves to place your stones in the most advantageous way. It takes a lot of concentration and study to play these games. It is like life's situations. Many times you need to look ahead to know where you are going. Our trip now is similar to the game you see in the painting."

Pei Ke started inwardly at his master's sudden reference to their current journey. Since they had left, he had said nothing directly about it, but Pei Ke had noticed him touching the message and looking thoughtfully at the trees and birds. Clearly something had happened that had disturbed the master.

Even as he wondered again at what the message said, he shook his head in admiration for his master's devotion to learning and wisdom. Even the games in life take study, he thought. Does the master ever have fun for the sake of having fun?

"Pei Ke, are you familiar with the I-Ching?"

"I have heard of it, of course. But my father was a simple man. He only believed in things immediately practical. Concepts like the I-Ching were beyond him. He only knew hard work."

"You should understand the philosophy of the I-Ching and the role it plays in our daily lives. It dates back more than two thousand years. Conflicting legends and historical information about the original work abound but most people believe that Emperor Wen first described it. Though its parameters may have changed since originally conceived, the essence of what it is remains intact."

Liu fiddled with his hands and slid each arm into the opposite sleeve. Pei Ke was impressed that Liu could take on the appearance of a martial arts master one moment and a scholar the next moment.

"Some historians believe that Confucius and Lao Tzu were both ardent students of the I-Ching, and the I-Ching had a direct influence on their philosophies. Others believe the I-Ching foretells the future. I have marveled at their ignorance for the I-Ching does not predict one's future. It is only a guide for one to consider in the course of one's life.

"Of course, I have an unusual theory and viewpoint about the I-Ching. We know that the universal Tao is composed of Yin and Yang. The sun is Yang and the earth is Yin. We know a continual interplay exits between Yin and Yang; they seem to balance each other. This Yin and Yang of the universe affects our weather, tides, life, death, and so forth. If we accept this theory of Yin and Yang, and what it means, we can accept the fact of the Universal Energy. This energy manifests itself in different ways. It surrounds our body and is part of our body. Our thought process is nothing more than bits and pieces of energy flowing in a stream. Our internal energy blends into the external energy surrounding us. So in essence, we as energy, blend in as part of the Universal Energy. This Universal Energy affects us just as we in some minute way affect the overall Universal Energy. The I-Ching helps us to make a connection between our energy and the Universal Energy through our thought process.

"If you think about a certain statement, it will cause your energy to manifest itself in a certain pattern. When you cast the Yarrow stalks or coins of the I-Ching your energy interacts at that moment with the Universal Energy, and the casting only tells you how you fit into that energy at that moment. As your life situations change from day to day, your energy with a particular statement will change as it interacts with the Universal Energy. Thus, the I-Ching is only a guide along a path. Whereas, some would say you are predetermined to do some things, I disagree, for I believe we all have free will. We can choose our destiny. The I-Ching is only our guide. It makes no decisions for us. We are free to choose or not to choose a course of action."

"Master, it means we have to accept the concept of energy."

"Why shouldn't you accept it? Why would you want to fight it? Take a moment and feel your emotions at this very minute. Now I want you to say to yourself 'I accept this philosophy of the Tao and the concept of energy,' and pay attention to how you feel physically, emotionally, and spiritually. After you have experienced this feeling I want you to say to yourself, 'I do not accept this philosophy of the Tao and the concept of energy' and see how you feel physically, emotionally, and spiritually."

Pei Ke did as instructed.

"Master, I sense a difference, but I cannot explain it."

"The ancients, because of their simple life, were more in tune with their energy. You can accept things and be at peace with yourself, or you reject things and always argue with yourself. It is your choice. Just remember to think of yourself as pure energy. Your body is only a means of storing this pure energy. When I was in Shanghai, I visited with some friends. They took me to hear a lecture by a Western religious person. In the West they have competing religions, each claiming to be the 'true' religion. They have come to China to convert our people to their religious beliefs. One of these religious people made an interesting statement. He said we were made in the image of God. Most of them believe there is only one god. If you believe the energy theory I have been describing, then he is entirely correct. He is correct but for reasons he does not know, nor will he ever know. Many religions and philosophies have come and gone. These religions, no matter what they are, are fine as long as they do not violate you as a human being. Any philosophy that does not respect human life should be avoided. Remember, however, that this is only my opinion and will probably be criticized by many others you will likely meet."

Pei Ke thought for a moment and was about to ask a question when Liu started speaking again.

"The ancients used a set of dried Yarrow stalks to cast the I-Ching. This is a complicated way of getting to an answer. An easier way, which will give somewhat the same answer, is to use three coins of the same size, weight, and shape and to cast these three coins six times and record each casting.

"Looking at the coins, you first need to determine which side is Yang and which side is Yin. Avoid confusion by using the side of the coin with the writing as the Yin side and the side without the writing as the Yang side. It makes no difference as long as you are consistent and can distinguish one side from another. The Yin side is given a value of two and the Yang side is given a value of three. Are you paying attention?"

"Yes, Master."

"You will need to remember what I am telling you."

"Yes, Master."

"Then think of a question. Keep the question to yourself since this is your energy. Consistently think of this question each of the six times you cast the coins.

"After throwing the coins, add up the value of the throws, which is the total of coins face up. Thus if two of the coins landed with writing face up, they would be Yin, and one was face up without writing, it would be Yang, and you would have a total of two plus two plus three, or seven. Since we are dealing with only the value of two and three the only possible totals are six, seven, eight, and nine. There are no other possible combinations.

"If the total adds up to six or eight the casting is considered Yin, which in this case is represented by a broken line. If the total of the casting is a seven or a nine, it is a Yang casting and is represented by an unbroken line. If the total is a six or nine, it is considered a changing line, since it would add up to all two's or all three's. If it is a changing line then a check mark will be placed next to the line to indicate it changes.

"Pei Ke, may I use three of your coins?"

"How did you know I am carrying coins?"

"I can hear them rattling in your pocket, and you are constantly checking to make sure they are still there."

Blushing yet again, Pei Ke reached inside his pants to the not-so hidden pocket and pulled out three small coins.

"Make sure there is writing only on one side of each coin. Some coins have writing on both sides."

Pei Ke looked at the three coins. They were of the same size, shape, and weight and each had writing only on one side.

"I want you to think of a question that is important to you, one for which you would like to have some direction. The question has to be one in which you are seeking guidance, not the accumulation of wealth. The question should also be ethical and not deal with the intention to harm anyone. Questions that start with 'Is it appropriate for me to do' would be fine for now. Do you have a question?"

"May I have more than one question?"

Liu shook his head, smiling inwardly.

"You and your questions. Just think of one question, Pei Ke, and put the rest from your mind."

Pei Ke looked at Liu and was about to ask another question, then thought it better not to ask.

"I am ready."

"Concentrate on the question and throw the coins on the table. Let's see what you get."

Pei Ke threw the coins. Two had visible writing and one had no writing.

"What did you get?"

"There is a two, a three, and a two, which means Yin, Yang, and Yin, right? That comes to a total of seven, which is Yang."

"That is correct. Is the line changing?"

"No, because the coins are not all Yin or all Yang."

"Good. Cast the coins five more times. We remember the tosses from bottom to top. So your next answer will be placed a little above the first answer."

Liu took a small piece of rice paper from the table and laid it flat. He touched one finger to his mouth and then to the paper. The saliva made a slight discoloration on the paper. He drew a line about one inch in length. On each succeeding throw, he would make a mark on the paper—either a solid line or a broken line—always making the mark above the preceding mark. He carefully noted the changing lines.

"Good. The only line that is changing is the last one."

"Is this good or bad?" asked Pei Ke.

"It is neither good nor bad. It depends on the question, and how you interpret the answer in light of the question."

Liu looked at the hexagram for a few minutes. Pei Ke sensed it was not a good time to ask any questions.

"In light of the question you asked, the throw of the coins gave you the third hexagram. There are a total of sixty-four possible hexagrams. The third hexagram of the I-Ching indicates there will be difficulty at the beginning. The top line had a changing process so the hexagram has totally changed and has become the forty-second hexagram, which is a further elaboration of the first hexagram. The forty-second hexagram indicates that there is an increase, which means the difficulty in the beginning may be increased. The implication is that the difficulty is longer than normal, but it is quite possible to overcome the difficulty and achieve what you had asked."

Pei Ke looked at Liu, dumbfounded. He had no idea what to say. The I-Ching was correct. He struggled constantly with what he wanted to do with his life and there was no end in sight to the conflict.

# MARKS THAT LIU PUT ON
# THE RICE PAPER

## COINS

Yin = 2

Yang = 3

Changing Line = 6 or 9

## TOTAL OF THREE COINS

Yin = 6 or 8 = broken line

Yang = 7 or 9 = unbroken line

## INITIAL THROW OF THE COINS

## WITH CHANGING LINES

| Throw | Results | Change | Changes |
|---|---|---|---|
| 6 | ▬▬▬  ▬▬▬ | < | ▬▬▬▬▬▬ |
| 5 | ▬▬▬▬▬▬ | | ▬▬▬▬▬▬ |
| 4 | ▬▬▬  ▬▬▬ | | ▬▬▬  ▬▬▬ |
| 3 | ▬▬▬  ▬▬▬ | | ▬▬▬  ▬▬▬ |
| 2 | ▬▬▬  ▬▬▬ | | ▬▬▬  ▬▬▬ |
| 1 | ▬▬▬▬▬▬ | | ▬▬▬▬▬▬ |

3

*Difficulty in the beginning*

42

*Increase*

# CHAPTER NINE

After leaving the teahouse, Liu Bin and Pei Ke traveled on their northerly course over the mountains. This was the first time Pei Ke had been this far from his village, and he was amazed to see the various differences, not only in the vegetation, but also in the dialect and mannerisms of the people he saw.

"Master?"

"Yes."

"We have talked about Yin and Yang, Blood and Qi but you have not told me about the Five Elements."

"What would you like to know?"

"I have heard about them and how they influence our life, of course, but all I really know is that they represent items in nature."

"You are partially correct, in that they represent concepts of nature but the idea is quite elaborate. The theory of Yin and Yang is older than the theory of the Five Elements. However, taken together they are the foundation for the development of Chinese medicine. Historians tell us that the first reference to the Five Elements theory goes back over two thousand years. Like most discoveries, the theory has undergone different stages of development. At times it was quite popular and other times it lost some of its importance and glamour. When you study the theory in more detail, you will understand why it is one of the cornerstones of the overall philosophy of the Chinese people."

"My parents were interested in the theory. They would mention it to me, but I was too busy having a good time to pay close attention."

"To say the Five Elements are really physical elements of nature is not truly correct. We need to use the words in a different sense. It would be better to refer to the Five Elements as the five phases, five processes, five stages, five patterns, five movements, or five qualities."

"Master, we all go through stages, events, and patterns in our lives. Is this what you are referring to as the Five Elements?"

"Yes, but there is more to it than that."

"Master, please explain."

"The Five Elements are Metal, Water, Wood, Fire and Earth. You should remember them in this order. Some philosophers have them in a different order, but that is for a later day and a later lesson, and so you should memorize them as I have said them.

"Each one of these elements represents a movement of nature. For example: metal is contractive, water is downward, wood is expanding in all directions, fire indicates upward trends, and earth represents the center. Furthermore, the elements can represent seasonal changes: Metal is associated with autumn, Water is associated with winter, Wood is associated with spring, Fire is associated with summer, and Earth is associated with late summer. Remember when I told you about Yin and Yang and how each meridian is either Yin or Yang?"

"Yes, Master."

"Well, each meridian is not only Yin and Yang, but is associated with one of the Five Elements. Metal is associated with Lung Meridian and Large Intestine Meridian."

"So each meridian is either Yin or Yang and each one of them is associated with one of the Five Elements?"

"Yes, They are associated with many different aspects of what we know, including not only the directions and seasons, but also colors, tastes, climates, human development, grains, sense organs, tissues, emotions, and sounds."

"What is the emotion for the Fire Element?"

"Is that important?"

"I remember my parents saying that I was fire."

"The emotion for Fire is joy and happiness. Are you an excessively joyful person or do you lack joy in your life? One is a positive aspect of the Fire Element and the other is a negative aspect of the Fire Element. Don't think of the positive and negative aspects as being good and bad; rather think of them as opposites."

"I don't think I'm overly joyful or lacking in joy. I'm just in the middle. Is that bad?"

"No, that is good. As you guessed, your energy is balanced in the aspect of the Fire Element. It is the person who is always excessively joyful or never joyful who is not balanced; and that means something is wrong with the Fire Element. Every day we go through changes in our body, so at any one moment we may be or show tendencies towards one or more of the elements. When we are stuck on one of the aspects of the Five Elements is when we start to have our problems in life."

"So it means if you know what emotion is unbalanced you can treat that element and see a change."

"In theory you are correct, but it is not always so simple."

"What is the element for anger?"

"Anger and depression are associated with liver and the element of Wood. The sequence you need to memorize is as follows:

"Metal is associated with lung and large intestine, a westerly direction, the season of autumn, the color white, a pungent taste, a dry climate, the season for harvesting, the sense organ nose, the body part which is skin, and the emotions of sadness and crying.

"The Water Element is associated with kidneys and urinary bladder, north, winter, black, salty, cold, storage, ears, bones, fear, and groaning.

"The Wood Element is associated with liver and gall bladder, east, spring, green, sour, wind, birth, eyes, sinews, anger, and shouting.

"The Fire Element is associated with heart and small intestine, south, summer, red, bitter, heat, growth, mouth, joy, and laughing.

"The Earth Element is associated with spleen and stomach, center, late summer, yellow, sweet, dampness, transformation, muscles, pensiveness and singing. It would be to your advantage to make a chart of these relationships. It will help you to memorize them.

"Knowing the relationships as I have described them above will help you in diagnosing a patient. For example, if a patient complains of a sour taste in his mouth, which of the Five Elements could possibly be involved?"

"A sour taste is associated with wood."

"Yes, not only is it associated with wood, but wood is the element of liver and gall bladder. Thus if someone has a sour taste in his mouth, you may want to consider that his problem exists with the liver and/or gall bladder. However, I want to caution you about jumping to a conclusion until you have done a complete differential diagnostic analysis."

"Master, would this mean that someone who has an ear problem, like ringing in the ears, could also have a kidney problem?"

"Yes, you are correct. It would be better to say the kidney energy is not correct than say there is a kidney problem. The reason is that the energy of the kidney goes to the ears and in its unbalanced nature can cause ringing in the ears. Just because the kidney energy is unbalanced does not mean the actual kidney organ is defective or diseased. Do you understand the difference?"

"Yes, Master, I think so."

"You need to be clear about this. Give it some thought and let me know later. The important thing to remember is that this is just one possibility. However, it is known that ringing in the ears can also be treated by using the Triple Warmer Meridian and the Small Intestine Meridian, since both of these Yang meridians connect with the ear."

This was easy, thought Pei Ke. All he had to do was memorize these relationships and he could become a doctor.

"Master?"

"Yes."

"It seems that it would be easy to diagnose a patient's problem by the use of the Five Elements. From what you indicate, a person would have a number of characteristics like strange tastes or smells. Maybe they have an unusual emotional state, or a problem with one of their sense organs. Knowing this information I could find out what internal organ and meridian are involved and treat the problem."

"You are on the right track, but you only have one small piece of the puzzle. You must be a better detective to be a good doctor. Our bodies are complex organisms. What affects one part of our body will invariably affect another part of our body. Based on our constitutional development we manifest our problems differently. For example, if your only clue was that the person had a sour taste in his mouth, what conclusion would you draw?"

"Master, that is easy. Based on what you told me, a sour taste means there is a problem with the Wood Element which means Liver Meridian and Gall Bladder Meridian."

"Good, you said meridian instead of organ. Pei Ke, have you ever had an upset stomach from eating food that wasn't clean, and later had a sour taste in your mouth?"

"Yes, Master."

"The sour taste from bad food might have nothing to do with your liver."

"Yes, Master."

"Ask the patient as many questions as possible to build a pattern that allows you to make the correct decision."

"Master...."

"Let me finish. Once you know the Five Elements, you must know that within our lives exists the generating and destructive sequence of the elements. You will memorize the generating or creative sequence of the Five Elements. Thus, metal will enhance water, water will enhance wood, wood will enhance fire, and fire will enhance earth. This is a continuous, never-ending cycle. The seasons follow this cycle; our birth, maturity, and death follows this cycle."

"I do not understand."

"You can use a metal shovel to dig for water. Thus, metal creates water. The water nourishes the tree. Thus, water creates wood. Wood makes a fire. Thus, wood creates fire. Fire creates ashes, which become part of the earth. Thus, fire creates earth. Earth creates metal. Earth is compressed and its weight creates metal. The cycle continues on one element creating or generating the next element in that particular pattern."

"Master, I know I should not ask too many questions, but in your example metal creates water. However, doesn't water destroy fire? We put out the campfire by means of water."

"Mentally draw a circle and place the Five Elements equidistant around the circle. In this circle of life, one element follows the other. Now skip every other element and you have the destructive or controlling sequence of the Five Elements. The destructive order would be metal, wood, earth, water and fire. In this sequence metal destroys wood similar to the ax cutting down the tree, wood destroys earth similar to the tree absorbing the nutrients from the earth, earth destroys water similar to when it rains and the water is absorbed into the earth, and water destroys fire similar to your example of putting out the campfire with water."

"Master, how do the two cycles of creating and destroying relate to healing?"

"We have different ways to use this information, but two primary methods exist. You can use the sequence of the elements to treat the patient or you can treat the patient according to the Five Transporting Points. Both methods are used. Clinical experience will be invaluable in deciding which one to use. Incidentally, many individuals prefer one method to the other and use it exclusively in their practice. In essence, they do Five Element acupuncture.

"Master which one do you use?"

"I do not limit myself to only one protocol. Neither does the accomplished doctor. There are many protocols to use in treating the patient. Your accumulated experience and learning helps you make a decision on how to treat the patient. I will tell you the many things I have learned from my teachers. You will decide what and how to use the information."

"Master, look out!" screamed Pei Ke.

Liu felt someone grab his left shoulder. From the distribution of the pressure and the location of his attacker's thumb, Liu knew the person used his right hand. Liu instantly stepped forward with his right foot, rotating his heel into the dirt to start a rooting process.

The moves in Tai Chi Chuan are graceful and beautiful and are done slowly to build up the internal energy, but no move in his style of Tai Chi Chuan could be executed without being rooted. Liu then turned his body to the left so he was at a right angle to the attacker. Two things happened. The distance between him and his opponent increased and the attacker was pulled slightly off balance, causing him to step forward with his right foot. Liu turned his waist to the left and shifted his weight to his right foot, allowing him to pick up his left foot.

He then hooked his left foot behind the heel of his attacker's right foot, preventing the attacker from withdrawing the foot. Liu shuffled to the right dragging his and the attacker's foot towards him. The attacker was off balance. Liu sensed the right knee joint and right leg muscles of his attacker were relaxed and vulnerable. He sat straight down into a strong but relaxed horse stance. As he sat into this move, his arms went to both sides, his shoulders opened forward slightly to give structural integrity to his body, and his left hand made contact with his attacker's right leg just above the knee. His thumb rested on a special acupuncture point dealing with Qi while his index finger fell on Xue Hai acupuncture point on the Spleen Meridian, which deals with blood. He applied swift downward pressure while simultaneously squeezing both acupuncture points.

The combination of downward pressure, squeezing the two acupuncture points and trapping, the right foot shut off the attacker's Qi and Blood. The attacker fainted and collapsed to the ground. The movement was over in a fraction of a second.

Pei Ke stared in amazement. He remembered himself wondering if the stories he had heard about Liu were true, but now he had seen it with his own eyes. His heart was racing and he was breathing heavily.

"Master, is he dead?"

"No, Pei Ke," said Liu. "He just feels a little weak. All of the fight has been taken out of him."

"How did you do that?" Pei Ke stared at the man now lying on the dirt road.

"Let's leave here before there is more trouble. I will explain later."

As they quickly moved away from the altercation, Pei Ke looked back to see the assailant slowly rising from the ground. He did not appear to be injured, just a little dazed and overwhelmed by the suddenness of the response to the attack.

How he wished he could do that and with such speed. The old master knew exactly what to do and how to do it. He touched the exact spots on the man's leg. Unlike the master, he would still be thinking about what to do and searching for the correct location.

He looked over at the older man, who was apparently deep in thought.

Liu did not recognize the man who had attacked him. It was possible he was just a bandit, but Liu did not believe so. He knew the conflict he had been sensing and this somehow seemed involved with it. He read through the message in his mind again, this time through the filter of this attack and he began to feel more unsettled about his family.

They walked quickly for the rest of the day and after several hours, Liu could no longer ignore his student, who continued to stare openly at him as they traveled.

"If you are wondering how I knew what to do, there is no secret. It requires a competent teacher, a dedicated student willing to listen and not ask too many questions, diligent practice, and strong legs. Many teachers of Tai Chi Chuan emphasize that the power of Tai Chi Chuan is due to the waist. They are correct but it is the ability to root to the earth which allows one to turn the waist."

"Master, who was the attacker? Why would he want to hurt you?"

"I suspect it has something to do with the note I received and my journey home."

"Should we go to the authorities?"

"No, it will only waste time. The assailant is gone. I don't think we will be bothered for the rest of the day."

"The rest of the day? Should we get some weapons?" asked Pei Ke.

"Do you know how to use a weapon?"

"No."

"Then the weapon is useless. Granted you might use it once to hold off the attacker for a minute, but an accomplished martial artist will penetrate your defense and take your weapon. Then he will use it against you."

Pei Ke wished he had kept his mouth shut.

# CHAPTER TEN

"Master?"

"Yes."

"We have been traveling for two days now. When will we get to your parents' home? How far is your family from the village?"

"I have already told you. We will travel many more days before we get to the village. If we hurry, tonight we will stay with Master Ling, one of my martial arts brothers. I have known him for many years, and he is a good friend of the family. He might be able to help us understand what has happened."

"I didn't know you had a martial arts brother. What style of martial arts does he practice?"

"He originally trained in the external martial arts as I did. His father first taught him Shaolin and then their family style of martial arts. . My father taught me our family's style of martial arts, which is different from Master Ling's style. There are hundreds of family styles of Chinese martial arts that are passed on from one generation to another. Some emphasize leg movements, while others emphasize hand movements. Regardless of what style is known, the origin of these styles was Shaolin. Shaolin is Buddhist in nature and taught exclusively to the Buddhist monks at the Shaolin temple.

"Family styles stay within the family. If the family line dies out, most likely the family martial art will be lost. The family martial arts are seldom taught to women. With the many revolutions in China, whole families and villages have been wiped out. There is always the sadness of loss of life, but there is also the sadness in the loss of a family's tradition.

"After practicing for years, Master Ling switched to the internal martial arts. He is very good in Hsing-Yi Chuan and Pa Kua Chang. We studied together for a couple of years. Our Hsing-Yi Chuan derives from the tradition of Master Kuo Yen Shen and the Pa Kua Chang derives from the tradition of Master Tong Hai Chuan.

"Hsing-Yi Chuan has a long history. It is reputed to have been founded by Yue Fei, a famous general in ancient times. Yue Fei developed the art so his soldiers would be invincible in battle. The lineage of Hsing-Yi Chuan is murky, however, and there are different versions.

"The most sensible version is that Yue Fei developed Hsing-Yi Chuan in the Sung Dynasty, and taught it to his troops. Their excellent training under Yue Fei allowed them to be victorious in battle. Yue Fei wrote a manuscript on the art. Some say it was lost. Others say it fell into the hands of an anonymous Taoist monk who later passed it on to Chi Lung Feng. Chi studied the manuscript and became a proficient teacher in the art. His most notable disciples were Ma Hsieh Li and Chao Chi Wu. Chao Chi Wu taught Tai Lung Pang who taught Li Lao Nan. Li Lao Nan taught Kuo Yun Shen. I learned the system as taught and modified by Kuo. This system includes the basic Five Elements of the art plus twelve animal styles.

"The Five Elements of Hsing-Yi Chuan are the same Five Elements of medicine. Here, each of the Five Elements refers to a particular basic martial art move within the Hsing-Yi Chuan system. The animal styles of Hsing-Yi Chuan incorporate the Five Elements into the fighting style of each animal."

"What are the animal styles of Hsing-Yi Chuan?" Pei Ke asked.

"It depends on the system of Hsing-Yi Chuan you have learned. Different teachers have incorporated different animals into their system. The system we practice includes the forms of chicken, horse, tiger, eagle, hawk, bear, turtle, Tai bird, dragon, monkey, snake, and swallow. In addition, some forms combine the various forms into one separate linking form. When you practice these animal styles within the Hsing-Yi Chuan system, each movement you execute should represent the movement of that particular animal. So when you watch someone practicing horse movements, it should actually look like a horse fighting."

"Which of the twelve animal styles do you prefer?"

"I do not have a favorite. I find the five basic postures of Hsing-Yi Chuan more important than the animal styles. If you truly master these five basic postures, you will be able to adequately defend yourself against most attacks."

"You mean all you need to know are the five basic postures of Hsing-Yi Chuan and you will be able to handle yourself?"

"Yes. The gifted Hsing-Yi Chuan masters can use these Five Element postures and variations on these postures to handle almost any situation. That is why the five basic postures need diligent practice. To develop the power of Hsing-Yi Chuan, you must practice standing in the San Ti posture for many hours. It is a very simple move when you first see it, but it is the cornerstone for developing power in the Hsing-Yi Chuan moves. You need to remember that. Many times students want to learn as much as possible and overlook what the old masters discovered."

"Did you personally know Kuo?"

"No, my martial arts brother and I learned from one of his top students."

"Did you study Pa Kua Chang from Master Tung Hai Chuan?"

"I learned Pa Kua Chang from one of his students."

"What do you know about Master Tung Hai Chuan?"

"I've heard different stories about Master Tung Hai Chuan. Many of his original students are alive today, and they have conflicting stories as to the origin. Tung told each one of them a bit of his history, but neglected to share everything with any one person. What we do know is that Master Tung was one of the first to publicly teach this art. I have heard this from more than one of his students. Some say he learned it from an anonymous Taoist monk. Others say he combined his previous knowledge and training in Shaolin with other martial arts to create this system. What we do know for sure is that he was born in the Wen An district of Hebei province."

"Did he teach many students?"

"According to my teacher, Master Tung taught over a hundred students, and had ten to twelve who excelled at it. The most famous were Cheng Ting Hua and Yin Fu. Of course, there were others, but these two have the most students. When you compare the Pa Kua Chang of Cheng Ting Hua and the Pa Kua Chang of Yin Fu you will see the differences, of course."

"Why is that?" asked Pei Ke.

"Most of Master Tung's students already knew a martial art when they came to him. Master Tung taught them differently since he based his teachings on what they already knew. Of course, each one then modified it to suit his individual martial arts strengths. So today, we have different styles of Pa Kua Chang, but the essence of Pa Kua Chang is the same for all the different styles. Pa Kua Chang is known for its circular movements which are practiced while walking a circle. Very quick turns allow you to circle your opponent. This coiling attribute allows the accumulation of coiling energy, a distinctive feature of Pa Kua Chang."

"When did you learn?"

"While living in Beijing. I had heard about this great martial art and wanted to see it for myself. I studied the art for three to four years. I devoted my entire day and night to it. You think I am good, but others are better than I am. Always remember, no matter how good you are, there is always someone better. Don't let your ego get in the way of knowing who you are or what you are capable of doing."

"Master, do you think I could learn Pa Kua Chang in four years?"

"You have to remember I had a good background in martial arts before I started with Pa Kua Chang. This background helped me to learn quickly. Many martial artists know more than one martial art. As an example, many of the martial arts practitioners of Hsing-Yi Chuan also know Pa Kua Chang."

"Why?"

"When you begin to gain a reputation in a particular martial art, you are often challenged by others to see how good you are. They don't want to hurt you, but rather they want to find out if your skills are as good as they have heard. They also want to see if their skills are good enough to defeat you. One day Kuo, the Hsing-Yi Chuan master, challenged Tung to a friendly competition. The competition went on for two days with neither winning. On the third day, Tung won the match. Some say he won because he was so much better and others claim they were evenly matched. When Kuo lost, he prostrated himself in front of Tung. It was his way of showing Tung that a superior martial artist had defeated him. The two of them later became friends and agreed that their students should study the other's art. It is difficult to believe Tung would do this unless he knew Kou had some exceptional skill. Today many of the Hsing-Yi Chuan masters have now studied Pa Kua Chang, and many of the Pa Kua Chang masters have studied Hsing-Yi Chuan. That is one of the reasons I went to Beijing to study Pa Kua Chang."

"Master, you have studied all three internal martial arts. In your opinion, which of the three is the most effective for self defense?"

"All Chinese martial arts are effective, regardless of whether it is one of the external martial arts of Hung Gar, Shaolin, Praying Mantis, Choi Le Fut, and so on, or the three internal martial arts. The practitioner makes the difference. The hard martial arts are best suited for the young, and the soft internal martial arts are best suited for those in later years. Each of the three internal martial arts has its own distinctive quality, lending itself to unique situations. I do not think any one of them is any better than another.

"It is the combination of the three, in the hands of the right practitioner, which makes for a comprehensive art. In essence, the three of them are all the same. However, for sheer directed force, Hsing-Yi Chuan is probably the most effective. The power generated and the application of the force can literally crush bones. That is what happened to Kuo. He had an altercation with someone and hit him hard enough to kill him. For that reason, he spent some time in jail.

"For moving around your opponent, Pa Kua Chang is the art of choice because of the quick stepping pattern. The yielding ability of Tai Chi Chuan is well known and would be appropriate for dissolving an attack."

"Master, is it possible for someone like me to learn all three at the same time?"

"Yes, it is possible, but it would be better to learn one then another. In your situation, you will learn all three arts in segments. You will learn a segment and practice it repeatedly. When you have mastered one segment, I will teach you another segment. You will continue to practice what you have mastered and I will add more material as you progress. I warn you again that this is a commitment of many years of continuous study. It is not something you take lightly. As you learn the martial arts, you also will learn medicine, calligraphy, painting, and poetry."

Pei Ke thought for a minute. "Master, does this mean I will be studying continuously for many years?"

"Yes, the rewards are great. You will have a treasure when you are older."

"Master?"

"Yes."

"Do you think that I will be able to make money teaching martial arts?"

"Some make money teaching."

"Do they make a lot?"

"Is that your primary focus on learning?"

"No."

"Then do not worry about it."

Pei Ke again thought to himself about how poor he had been all his life. At times he had not known if he would have food, let alone a place to sleep. Did he really want to be poor forever? His parents were poor. His relatives were poor and he was destined to be poor if he followed in the footsteps of his teacher.

That evening just before sunset, they arrived at Master Ling's home. It stood in stark contrast to Mr. Wang's wealth and the teahouse. Ling lived as a hermit in a two-room, wooden shack next to a small, clear-water creek. In the background, mountains rose majestically.

Ling was about the same age as Liu and about the same build. His graying hair hung to his shoulders and his long eyebrows touched his ears and cheeks. This combination of long hair and eyebrows gave him the appearance of an old sage. His penetrating stare made Pei Ke shiver. If anyone ever fought with Ling, that stare alone could win the fight.

Pei Ke found it strange that the two men seemed to enjoy each other's company even though they said nothing of substance to each other. Liu got along with Ling as well as he had with Wang. In Pei Ke's mind, Liu did not make a distinction between the two individuals even though the men were obviously from different classes. Liu inquired about Ling's teaching and they immediately switched to a dialect that Pei Ke had not heard before. Pei Ke thought Ling was telling Liu about a group of men they both knew.

After dinner, the conversation continued between the two martial arts brothers. During a pause Pei Ke fell asleep.

He was not sure why he awoke, but when he did, the two men were gone. As he looked around, he heard faint sounds from outside. He hesitantly peeked through the shutter to see Liu and Ling in what appeared to be a friendly sparing match.

He was amazed to see their agility. The moonlight illuminated them. Each anticipated the other's move. Pei Ke thought he could see the Pa Kua Chang moves and the Hsing Yi Chuan moves based on what the master had told him. Other moves looked interesting, but he had no idea from what martial art they came. Even though the two men had trained with each other many years ago, there was a distinct difference in their styles. Ling was more aggressive than Liu. He was always on the offensive. But Liu had more finesse.

Pei Ke watched the men for more than an hour as each tried to outdo the other. They would come together, exchange a series of attacks, blocks, and counter attacks. Then they would separate for a few minutes to rest and analyze each other. No words passed between them. Pei Ke marveled that the two elders could continue without extended periods of rest. The men's show of power, speed and agility was unbelievable.

By the time he gave up and returned to his bed, Pei Ke's was forced to admit that the match would likely be a draw, though as he was falling asleep, he smiled as he thought of his master returning to the house victorious.

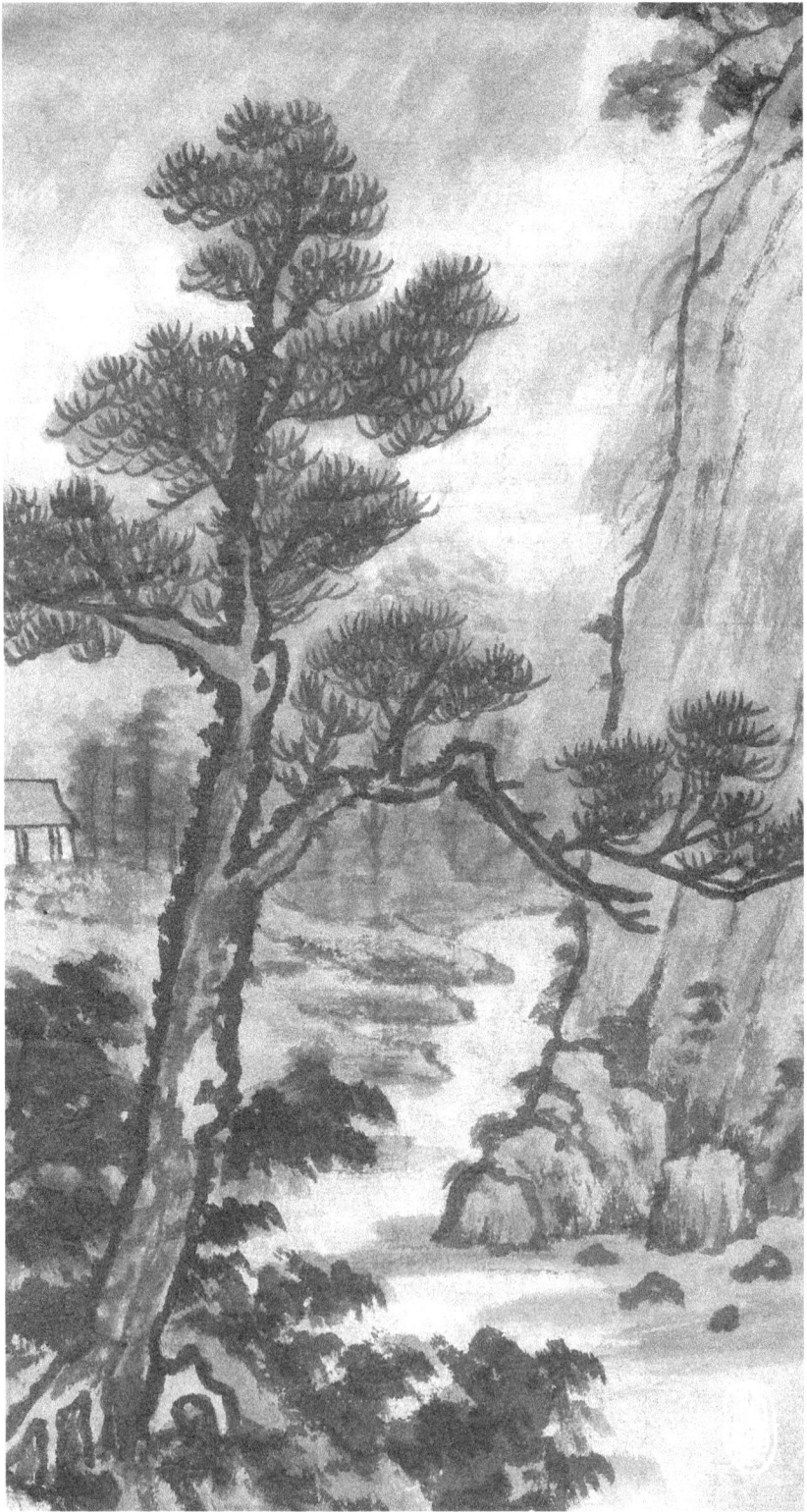

# CHAPTER ELEVEN

As Liu and Pei Ke walked along the road, Pei Ke followed Liu's instructions and felt his left wrist for the pulses. At first, the pulses seemed exaggerated, but as he moved his fingers over the radial artery, he could tell they were not exaggerated, but different than what they were before.

"Master, as I walk my pulses are faster, but there is also another difference. Why is that?"

"The pulses are changing for two reasons. First, as you walk your heart beats faster to get more Qi to the muscles so they can work appropriately. Without the flow of Qi, the muscles will not respond. Second, as you walk the imbalances along the meridians in your body tend to be momentarily corrected. When you stop walking, the pulses will return to where they were before. Those who exercise regularly will find that their pulses permanently change from an unbalanced state to a more balanced one. That is why those who practice martial arts such as Tai Chi Chuan, Pa Kua Chang, and Hsing-Yi Chuan on a regular basis have far fewer health care issues than those who do not.

"Actually, practicing Tai Chi Chuan will go a long way in reducing or preventing arthritis, high blood pressure, strokes, and heart attacks. As you practice, there will be less need for visits to the doctor. In addition, you will have an overall feeling of well being, though you may find that this feeling is hard to describe. I have taught Tai Chi Chuan to many elderly people and have found that when they practice on a regular basis, they fall less often, feel stronger, are more agile, sleep better, have fewer tremors, walk steadier, and are mentally more alert. They are far less inclined to have degenerative diseases.

"Regular practice of Tai Chi Chuan is one of the secrets of a long, healthy, and productive life. It is never too late to start, as long as you have an experienced teacher who is knowledgeable in the arts. These teachers are hard to find.

"Just remember: everything in moderation. As an example, too much exercise, done too quickly, can cause significant injuries to the body. As the body adapts and the Qi flows more evenly, then the body can handle an increase in exercise."

"Master, for someone like yourself, who seems to be in perfect health, is there such a thing as too much exercise?"

"The life cycle of a person determines a lot of what that person should and should not be doing. When one is young and the Qi is flowing abundantly, more exercise is appropriate. When one is elderly and frail, sitting exercises are probably all one can do. Even sitting exercise would be of some benefit."

"Can you do Tai Chi Chuan and Qi Gong while sitting? I thought that they had to be done standing and moving."

"It is possible to do both while sitting. Of course, you would get more benefit if you did it standing. At the beginning some people can only exercise sitting, but with time and practice, they can once again stand and move around unassisted. Tai Chi Chuan is a universal gift available to everyone. You only have to take advantage of it."

"Master, why don't more people learn Tai Chi Chuan, Pa Kua Chang, and Hsing-Yi Chuan?"

"It is difficult to find a qualified teacher. Many profess to know, but you need to find someone willing to pass on his knowledge. If you find such a teacher, you have found a real treasure."

Pei Ke thought for a moment about how lucky he was to have found Liu. Undoubtedly, Liu was a real treasure and Pei Ke needed to study as diligently as possible.

# CHAPTER TWELVE

Liu and Pei Ke continued the journey northward, covering twenty to thirty miles a day, depending on the terrain. The pain and tiredness which Pei Ke experienced the first couple of days faded from him. Each day brought a marvelous array of new sights, sounds and even unique smells

For Liu, the journey only magnified his uneasiness. The question of why he had received the note and what had happened to his family weighed heavily on his mind.

In addition, they were still being followed. Clearly Wang's man was not as effective as he had hoped. He had no doubt that he could handle things if they were attacked, but the implications of these sinister elements were unsettling. He found that he was grateful for Pei Ke's presence and inquisitive nature. It gave him the opportunity to focus his energy and attention on something over which he had some control.

They rose early each morning, regardless of where they were staying, and did a little Qi Gong to prepare themselves for the day's journey. They were fortunate to stay at a couple of monasteries along the route.

The monks knew of Liu and all welcomed him and Pei Ke. In exchange for giving them food and shelter for the night, Liu would minister to their health needs. The monks expressed their gratefulness, for they all realized his unique ability as a true healer. Pei Ke always helped with the menial chores of chopping wood or carrying water and he marveled that in the countryside, the monastery was never located close to a water supply. Pei Ke had heard his master talk enough about the importance of leg strength. As he trudged along with the water buckets suspended from a pole, he wondered if such had been the motivation for the lengthy chore.

In the monasteries, they always ate bland vegetables and Pei Ke never felt full after a meal. He wondered why the monks never prepared enough food to fill him up. No wonder the monks were all thin.

When they could not stay with the monks, they found shelter and food from someone in the countryside. Liu dressed like a monk and with his shaved head he had the appearance of a true monk. They always worked for their meals and lodging and Pei Ke soon got over the embarrassment of having to ask to stay for the night. Usually, as they traveled and needed food and water, a situation arose to provide for their needs. It was as if the universal energy knew they were hungry or tired and directed someone to be there to help them. Even though Pei Ke was weary at the end of each day of traveling, it was a peaceful, worry-free tiredness. He did not think the same was true for his master.

The farther north they traveled, the quicker Liu's pace became. When the terrain was level or sloped downward, Liu would walk at a brisk pace. As always, Pei Ke marveled at the strength and endurance of such an old man. Once, Pei Ke asked his master about their urgency, but his question was diverted by a review of the meridians.

As they walked they saw farmers toiling in the fields. It must be rewarding, thought Pei Ke, to have the gift to grow something. The farmers were not wealthy, but they appeared contented and happy. Young children were playing as children usually do. Chickens, pigs, and water buffalo were abundant. Everyone seemed adequately fed, healthy and without worries.

On the fourth day, they walked up a slight incline and Liu immediately stopped. He said nothing, but indicated for Pei Ke to stay where he was on the road. Then he disappeared into the woods. A few minutes later, he returned with a long straight piece of bamboo. Pei Ke looked questioningly at the master, waiting for an explanation, but the old man turned without a word and motioned for them to continue. Liu slowed his pace as they continued up the incline. Pei Ke was amazed to see a large river just ahead.

"Pei Ke, this is one of the largest rivers in this province and there are three ways to cross it. The first is to swim, but the current is very strong and the water is very cold this time of the year. The second is to go upstream many miles to where there is a walking bridge across a narrow part of the river. If we go to the walking bridge it will add two to three days to our journey and it should be clear to you now that we do not have time for such a detour. The third way is to cross here, but to do so, we must hire a boat. The trouble is that robbers own the boats. They will not allow anyone to cross without payment of some type. If they know you have money, they will take it, along with your belongings. Or they will promise to take you for a reasonable price, but once you are halfway across, they will threaten to throw you into the river unless you pay more money. Of course, most people will pay the price, which is usually very high. The current is very swift in the middle. Travelers who are in a hurry have no choice but to pay the extra amount. The boat owners will know I have no money, but they will suspect you have money. If they search the sack you are carrying, they will take whatever they want."

"Master, I cannot swim. If they throw me into the water I will drown."

"This is exactly their hope. Many who live in this area cannot swim. The lakes and rivers are too cold for most people and few get the chance to learn. I was fortunate to learn when traveling to the coast. But the men in the boat are hoping we cannot swim. When we get to the boat, let me do all the talking. Is that clear?"

"Yes, Master."

They continued to the river. When they arrived at the dock, Liu bowed to the two men. Liu knew there were more than just the two men with the boat. At least two and maybe three waited on the other side of the river, and at least one or two more hid out of sight on this side of the river.

"We would be indebted if you could help us cross the river," said Liu.

"It is one teal for each of you or you can go upstream and cross at the foot bridge," said the tallest and heaviest of the two.

"I do not have any money, but I would be willing to help you work or tell your fortune for safe passage."

Both men laughed, and the one who seemed to be in charge moved forward. "We don't need our fortunes told. Now, monk, pay or leave."

"What is the least you will charge us to get to the other side?"

"Half a teal is the lowest I will go, but only because you are a monk."

"Would that be for both of us?"

"For as many as will fit in the boat. The more the better, so I only have to cross one time."

"What is in the sack?" the other man said. He motioned to Pei Ke.

"The sack belongs to me and has personal things of value only to us. We will be back when we can," Liu said as he turned and walked back toward the direction they came from. Pei Ke followed without saying a word.

When they were over the rise on the other side of the incline, Liu stopped. "We will wait here for a little while."

"Why are we waiting?"

"We are waiting for more travelers. The boat will take maybe five passengers, plus two men to work the oars and steer the boat."

"Master, why aren't there honest men with boats so everyone has a choice of whom to use?"

"Fear, probably. We will wait for more travelers and maybe join up with them. Let's get off the road and wait in the forest."

"Why?"

"I want to see who is following us."

Pei Ke turned to look in all directions but saw no one.

"Master, how do you know they are behind us?"

"One or more of them have always been behind us. You just didn't pay attention."

"Why didn't you tell me?"

"What would you have done besides worry? Every five minutes you would have turned around to see if anyone was behind you. It would be obvious you knew you were being followed."

Pei Ke opened his mouth, but found nothing to say.

From this vantage point in the forest, Liu could see far down the road and up to the top of the incline. An hour passed, then two hours and still no travelers came by. The two men sat in silence. Suddenly Liu stood up and motioned for Pei Ke to follow. Two travelers came down the incline from the river. They had obviously come across the river by way of the boats. Liu walked to the middle of the road and Pei Ke followed. The two travelers were startled to see what appeared to be a monk emerging from the forest.

"We have no more money," said one of the travelers. "They charged us three times what is fair and then they charged us again in the middle of the river. If you want money, go and get it from those boat people. They are crooks."

"I don't want your money. These people with the boats, do you know who they are?"

Both men shook their heads, too afraid to say anything. They just stared at Liu and Pei Ke. They did not know whether to stay or run.

"I know they have taken your money unjustly. They wanted to charge us also, so we cannot get across the river. When you came across the river, were there one or two men in the boat with you?"

One of the men raised two fingers.

"Was anyone left on the shore when you came over to this side?"

Both men shrugged their shoulders in unison.

"How many are now on this side of the river?"

The man who had spoken looked at Liu for the longest time without saying anything, then finally spoke.

"There are four on this side of the river, I think. We did not see anyone else on that side. They might be over there, but we did not see them. If you are a monk, you probably do not have any money. How are you going to get to the other side?"

"Do these men have any weapons?" Liu asked.

"We did not see any, but they could have concealed weapons in their clothes."

"You are right," Liu said. "I personally do not have any money, nor do I seek riches. My family needs me, and I must get home as soon as possible. I rely on the kindness of others to help me."

The man looked around to make sure that no one was watching and reached into his shoe. "Here is one coin. Maybe they will let a poor monk cross for this coin."

Liu took the coin, bowed to both of the men, and they walked away quickly.

Pei Ke thought for a moment. Why would strangers give money to a monk? Maybe it was their way of giving a sacrifice to the gods, since the monks were supposed to be closer to the gods because of their prayer and sacrifice.

Liu turned and looked suddenly into the forest. Pei Ke looked in the same direction but did not see what Liu saw.

Liu was suddenly overcome with a sense of evil energy. The men who were following them were in the forest now, watching them. Good energy was pure and uplifting and gives one a sense and feeling of lightness. This energy he felt coming from the forest was heavy and oppressive, with feelings of greed and sinfulness. He wanted no part of it, but knew in his heart that very soon he would have to deal with it in a way that would be distasteful to him.

"Come," he said quietly to his student and he and Pei Ke turned and walked toward the boats.

"Master, I thought we were going to wait for some travelers to come our way and join with them to cross the river?"

"I have changed my mind. An opportunity has presented itself. The gods have seen our predicament and have opened a way for us to cross the river without wasting more time. We will take advantage of it now. Again let me do all the talking and pay attention. I might need your help."

They walked down to the two boats and the four men. Liu saw that the two from the other side were big and muscular. Their size alone would intimidate travelers. If these men threatened travelers in the middle of the river, most people would gladly give their money to these crooks to save their lives.

"You two are back. Do you have money to cross the river?"

"Yes, we have money. We do not want to waste any more time. Earlier we agreed on one-half teal to get us safely across the river."

"Yes. Are you ready?"

"Are there any other charges?"

"No. Just give us the money and we can go."

"You will get us across safely?"

"We've been doing this for many years. All our passengers have gotten across safely."

"How do I know you will do what you say you will do?"

"Again, we've been doing this for many years and have many satisfied customers. They are always happy when they get to the other side."

"We will pay you one half teal when we get to the middle of the river. I think that is fair."

The man looked at Liu and then at Pei Ke and thought for a minute. He did not seem used to such an inquisitive and shrewd passenger.

"Get in the boat."

One of the men from the opposite bank got in the boat, followed by Liu and Pei Ke, and finally the last man. Liu put his walking stick on the deck. The boat was typical of boats in that area. The flat, wide bottom allowed someone to stand and walk from bow to stern without capsizing the boat. Liu judged the boat to be twenty feet long, with seats for at least eight people. It would be difficult for one person to handle the boat. Two people made it easier, as each would paddle—one in the front and the other in the back. If there was an exceptionally strong current, a third person would steer. Today, the current, while moving quite swiftly, was not overly strong and two men could handle the current by manipulating the oars.

As they moved onto the river, everyone was quiet. Pei Ke marveled at the river's length and width. He and Liu had crossed other rivers and streams but none like this one. He turned and looked back at the shore and saw that there were now four men instead of two. He shivered and wondered if these were the men Liu thought were following them. He wondered if the river men would try and swindle them as well, or if there was some unspoken honor between nefarious scoundrels.

On some unheard cue, both men stopped rowing and the vessel started drifting down stream.

"We are half way and now it is time to pay for the trip." Both men stood up. "We know you have money so the price has changed to two teals. One teal is the price for each of you. If you don't give us the money, we are going to throw you into the river." The other man chuckled and Pei Ke shivered again.

Liu turned to the man that was behind him. "You agreed on one half teal for both of us."

"I changed my mind. Give me the money."

Liu reached into his pocket and took out one teal. "I will give you one teal for both of us, and no more. That is a lot of money for so little work on your part."

"We know you have more money than that. Now give us the money."

"Here is one teal." Liu stretched out his hand to give the money to the man in the stern of the boat. The man stepped forward and grabbed Liu's wrist and was about to twist it into a submission hold, but Liu suddenly brought his hand towards his body throwing the man off balance. The master then twisted his elbow up, over, and underneath the bandit's arm, throwing him off balance and into the water. Liu immediately picked up the bamboo pole he had brought with him and thrust it forward into the chest of the man who was in the bow. He too fell into the water with a yelp of surprise.

"Pei Ke, grab the forward oars and start rowing for the shore."

Pei Ke was caught totally off guard by his master's sudden aggressiveness, but the men were shouting and cursing swimming toward the boat. With a speed that made Liu proud, Pei Ke jumped forward and took the oars and started awkwardly rowing the boat. Liu was doing the same.

"You need to put the tip of both oars into the water at the same time and pull hard. Be sure and not simply skim the oar across the water. Row fast, so they do not catch us."

Pei Ke rowed quickly and saw that they were pulling ahead of the two men in the water. Ten minutes later, they were on the opposite shore. Liu pulled the boat ashore and placed the coin on the bow of the boat. He had kept his part of the bargain. Then they walked off at a brisk pace to distance themselves from the altercation.

Liu sensed the energy on this side of the river was very different from the energy on the far side and it reinvigorated him. They had lost some time, but could make it up if they walked a little faster.

"Master, do you think those men in the water will be all right?"

"My guess is they are good swimmers. They will have no problem getting back to the boat, but they will not forget this encounter and so the next time we travel this way we will need to take the foot bridge."

"Do you think they ever let anyone pass free?"

"Probably not," Liu said. "Sometimes the strong prey on the weak. The weak attract the strong."

Something in the way he said this last statement made Pei Ke feel that his master was not talking about the incident with the river bandits. There was a heaviness to his master's voice. In an effort to bolster Master Liu's spirits, he said, "But you are not as strong as they, yet you were able to easily defeat them."

Liu smiled.

"I had an advantage they were not aware of. In essence, I was stronger and they were weaker. You are weak now, but train your body and mind to be strong. You will not have to fear the strength of others when they want to impose their will on you."

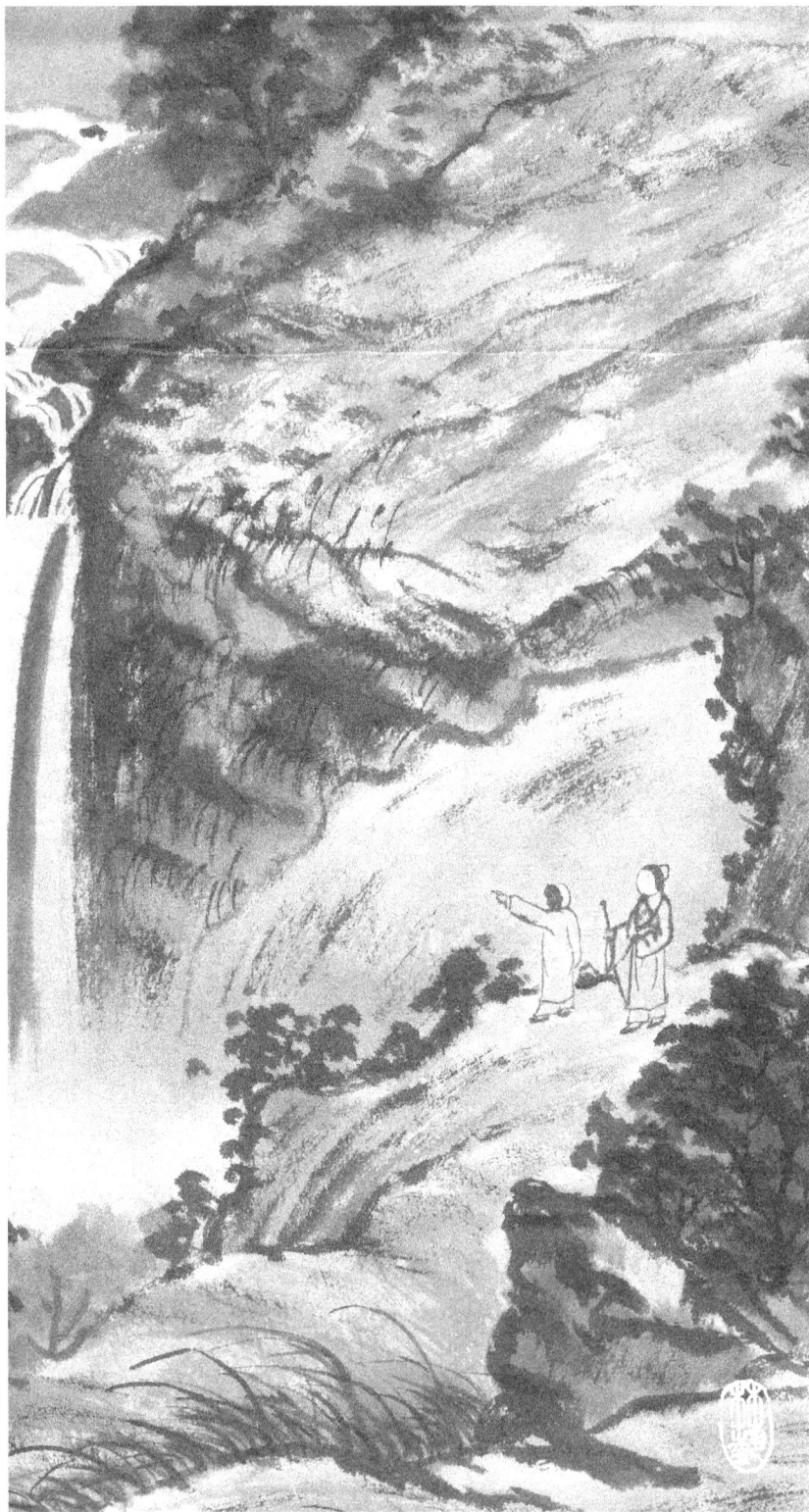

# CHAPTER THIRTEEN

On the fifth day they came upon a broad, flat plain dotted with many farms. Pei Ke could see that the fertile land provided an adequate living for the local inhabitants. This would be an ideal place to live, he thought. After a few hours of walking he sensed that the terrain was gradually sloping upward toward the distant mountains. As they left the farm area, they saw off to their left a large grove of mature trees surrounded by grassland.

As they walked, Pei Ke continued to ask questions, often jumping from martial arts to medicine and back to martial arts. On this particular day, he walked in a modified erect position, with legs slightly bent with his palms level with the ground. The energy on the Lao Gong acupuncture point was increasing and spreading through his arms and chest. He could also feel a tremendous energy rising up through his legs into his body from the acupuncture point Yong Quan. His legs hurt, but the energy more than made up for the pain. He was becoming addicted to the energy, and he knew it. He was becoming euphoric.

Suddenly they heard the sound of galloping horses. Pei Ke and Liu both looked at the forest area to their left and saw a large band of horsemen emerging from the trees. They were obviously heading in their direction.

"Pei Ke, when they arrive, I will do the talking. Only speak if you have no other choice."

"Master, do you know these soldiers?"

"No, but I know what they want. They are probably in this area to conscript men into the army."

Pei Ke's euphoria was swallowed by panic. He did not always know what he wanted out of his life, but he knew he did not want to be forced into the army.

"Master, should we run?"

He turned to run but Liu grabbed his shirt.

"Can you outrun a horse?"

As the soldiers drew closer, Liu recognized the banner of the Imperial Army and he counted thirty men. He knew if thirty came for two travelers, there must be a larger contingent inside the forest. He was surprised they would send so many men for just two people.

The troops drew abreast of Liu and Pei Ke. The leader signaled to the horsemen and they formed a mounted circle around the two travelers.

"Who are you?" asked the leader of the group.

"My name is Liu Bin and this is Pei Ke. We are poor travelers heading north to visit relatives."

"Are you a monk?"

"No, I am not a monk; but, I spend most of my time with them."

"Take the younger one, and let's go," the commander said.

Three men started to dismount.

"Wait," said Liu. "We travel together. Take us both."

The commander looked at Liu and Pei Ke, trying to make up his mind. There was something about Liu that made him unique, but he couldn't quite identify the feeling.

"Take them both," said the commander.

The three men, now dismounted, grabbed Liu and Pei Ke and pushed them in the direction of the forest.

"You can't outrun us," said one of the soldiers. "If you go peacefully you can walk on your own. If you resist or cause any trouble, we will chain you up and drag you."

"We will walk peacefully and not cause you any trouble," Liu said.

The commander and the rest of the contingent returned quickly to the forest. The three guards mounted and pointed in the direction of the forest. Liu and Pei Ke started walking with the soldiers following behind.

"Master, you could have defeated some of these men."

"Yes, I could have defeated some of them. But it is not possible to fight off thirty armed men on horseback and still protect you. Sometimes in life, it is much easier to take the road that has less force, to not meet force with force. This is Taoist philosophy. Let us see what they want of us."

Weeds clogged the dirt path. Pei Ke turned a couple of times, wishing the soldiers would disappear. His feeling of panic had subsided some but his stomach felt queasy.

A hundred feet into the forest, they came to a large clearing. In the center, the flag of the Imperial Army flew next to a large tent. Hundreds of smaller tents were neatly arranged around this the main tent. Pei Ke looked around in amazement that such an encampment could be so masterfully concealed so near the road.

Once in the encampment, they were led to the main tent.

———————

"I am General Tsu; I am in charge of this army unit. My commander tells me you are Liu Bin. Seldom is there an opportunity to meet new volunteers, but my second in command thinks there is something special about you and your friend. It is unusual to see an old man like you traveling in this part of the land. Where are you from?"

"My family is north in the mountains, about ten days walk from here."

"If your family is north of here, what are you doing in this area?"

"I live at a temple a few days south of here. I live with the monks and help them with chores."

"Who is this fellow?"

"His name is Pei Ke. He is one of my students. I feel I should tell you that you are now living on borrowed time. I could have easily killed you in the last thirty seconds. You have brought us here to conscript us into the army, but I want you to let us leave unharmed. In return, I will do you a favor. But I must have your word you will let us go."

The general looked startled and was about to call for the guards. Pei Ke was startled too. Had his master just threatened a general in the Imperial Army?

He saw Liu's right hand rise upward with the palm facing outward. At this, the general's face grew tight, as though he could not breathe or speak. He stiffened and fear filled his eyes, but then Master Liu lowered his hand and the general took a step forward, clutching at his throat and gasping for air.

"If you call for the guards, you will not live to see them," Liu said.

General Tsu looked toward the entrance to his tent. He looked back at Liu. Pei Ke did the same. The guards were only seconds away, but by what Pei Ke had just seen, the general could be dead in less than that if the master chose it.

"You said you would do me a favor if I let you go," the general said warily.

"First, I will let you live. Second, I see by the way you hold your arm you probably have severe shoulder pain and that you have had this pain for a long time. If you don't take care of it soon, it will become chronic and impossible to fix."

"Are you a doctor?"

"Yes, I am a doctor. I serve the monks in the temple where I live."

"We need doctors here with my men. Why don't you stay and help us?"

"No, I must be on my way to see my family. I have not seen them in many years."

The general looked at Liu and then Pei Ke.

"How do I know you will help fix my shoulder?"

"How do I know you will let both of us go? If my intent was to kill you, you would have already been dead. It is not worth losing your life and the lives of the other men in hopes of keeping us here."

"Fix my shoulder and you will be free to go."

"You mean both of us will be free to go?"

"Yes."

"Stand with your back straight and place your hands alongside your body."

Liu instructed the general on how to do quiet standing, which Pei Ke now knew was part of Qi Gong exercises. Within minutes, Liu sensed the general was a good receptor for the energy. Liu focused all his meditative ability on the general's right shoulder.

"What do you feel?" asked Liu.

"At first, I felt nothing, but now I feel this overall warming of my right shoulder and the pain is going away."

Pei Ke was amazed at what he saw. He felt the energy himself. His body warmed up. He looked at the general who was still standing in the Qi Gong position. The general was perspiring.

"How is the shoulder now?" Liu asked. "You can move it."

The general gingerly moved his right shoulder. As he moved his arm, he looked amazed and as he looked at Liu, greed came to his eyes. Liu understood. A man who could heal as he did would be invaluable to the army. He did not like acting aggressively but he needed to be moving on. His family could not wait for the whims of this general.

Before the man could even open his mouth for the guards, Liu stepped forward and the general's greed gave way to fear.

"How do you do what you do?" the general asked.

"I have been practicing martial arts and Qi Gong most of my life. There is nothing mystical about what I do. It is all learned techniques passed on from master to student."

"Your student is very lucky."

Pei Ke agreed silently.

Wearily, the general walked past Liu to the opening of the tent. Liu and Pei Ke followed him outside. The general walked over to where his commander was sitting.

"Take these two to the road. They are of no use to us."

———————

"Master, will you teach me how to do what you just did to the general?" Pei Ke asked when they were on their way again. "The man was impressed, thankful, and frightened all at the same time."

"You have too many questions," the master said. Then he quickened his pace again and Pei Ke had to almost run to keep up.

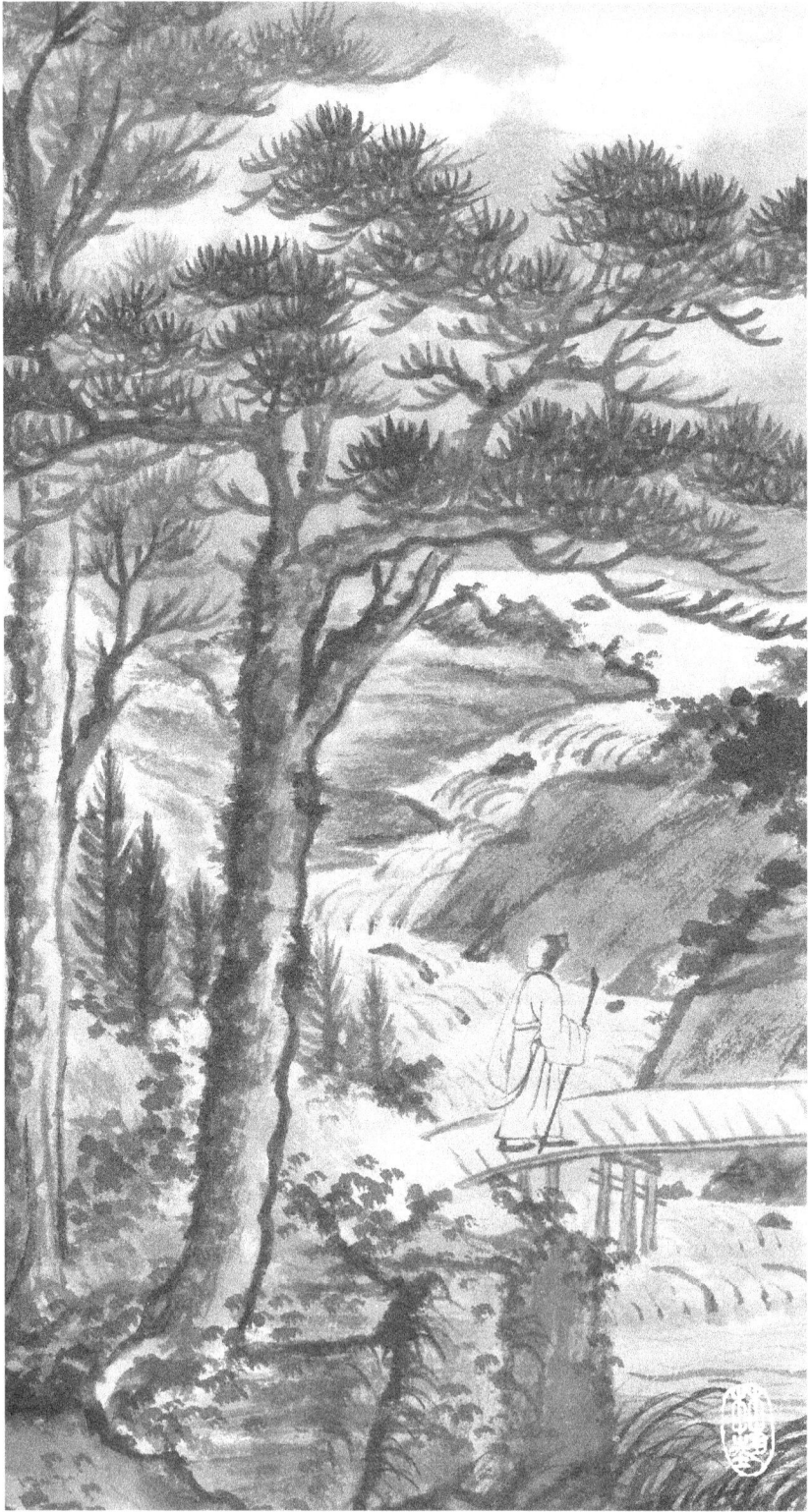

# CHAPTER FOURTEEN

For Pei Ke, every day presented a new and exciting learning experience. He not only continued learning martial arts, but also enhanced his knowledge of Chinese medicine.

The people he saw and the dialects he heard were an education in themselves. He felt lucky to be with Master Liu. Most people in rural China were born in, were reared in, and spent their entire lives in one small area. They never experienced what the country had to offer. They would never see the wide rivers, mountains with majestic views, and countryside lush with vegetation.

As Liu had indicated, most people were decent to them because he and Liu had been friendly to those they met. But, local people had no experience with travelers, and many were wary of strangers. As they entered the next village, Master Liu spoke again.

"Pei Ke, next we will visit an old friend. He will offer guidance as to what lies ahead. You will find him interesting. I first met him when I was a child. Fortune kept our paths crossing, and we became friends. He trained as a Taoist monk and now lives with other monks. Maybe he can help us understand why we are being followed."

Pei Ke looked behind them, but saw no one.

"Master, are they still following us?"

"Only one is following us now, but I sense others are involved."

"What happened to the other one?"

"I believe that Master Ling might have helped us out."

Pei Ke wondered if that person was still alive. He knew Master would never hurt anyone because it was against his religion and philosophy, but others were not so righteous. Pei Ke decided to keep the question to himself.

The village was not any different from others they had seen. A marketplace was still the village center and a couple of roads led out from its core. Most of the outlying farmers brought items to sell at the market. Here the basic items of trade were different from the south. Wheat and wheat products were readily available. Some farmers sold some rice, but Pei Ke could see that it was expensive in comparison to the wheat. Chicken and pork were the main sources of protein. Fish, unless it came from the rivers, was almost impossible to find. Occasionally, one found goat meat in one of the market stalls, but usually that meat was tough and suitable only for soup. The main vegetables were cabbage, Bok Choi, broccoli, and dried mushrooms. Pei Ke saw items he had never seen before, and he made a mental note to ask Liu if they could try some of the local delicacies before they left the village.

The owners of the vegetable and fruit stalls looked strangely at Pei Ke. They seemed to recognize some characteristic in him that was familiar to them. He was similar yet different. Maybe it was his facial features, or his height that set him apart. He was not as tall as most men in the village. His clothes were different, too.

"Pei Ke, pay attention and follow me. We will be going to a Taoist temple to see my friend. Please just listen."

"Yes, Master."

"Also," Liu continued, "for the time being we shall dispense with formality. I prefer that while we are here in the village, everyone just knows us as two travelers and not as teacher and student."

Liu turned off the main area of the village and headed down a small alleyway. Gates lined both sides of the long, crooked alley, each leading to a house. From the appearance of the gates and the condition of the wall, one had the impression that nothing of value was inside. However, Pei Ke knew differently. He looked up to the top of the walls and saw sharp pieces of metal and glass imbedded into the ledges. Once he heard a dog bark savagely at them from behind a gate.

One-story and two-story houses lined both sides of the crooked alley. The crookedness of the alley was determined by the Feng Shui of the building. The wanderings of the alley gave the impression of a dragon stretched out to the far corners of the village.

A whiff of smelly tofu caught Pei Ke by surprise. It was one of his favorite foods. One could easily recognize the odor of smelly tofu even from a great distance. It's distinctive odor was due to an additional fermentation process used in making this type of tofu. Pei Ke smelled it a block away. It smelled very bad, but it tasted unbelievably good. He had not had any of his favorite tofu since they started their long journey.

Liu stopped to read the signs posted on the walls of the alley. Throughout China the local villagers posted messages or notices on the outside walls. Old posters were always replaced with newer ones. Therefore, there were posters upon posters. Liu scanned the more recent additions.

Pei Ke wondered what Liu was looking for. Mostly, the posters only listed things for sale.

Liu pointed to one of the posters glued to the wall. Pei Ke turned to look at it and was amazed at the likeness of his master on the poster. He gasped as he realized its implication.

"Master…"

"Pei Ke…"

Pei Ke turned and saw the expression on Liu's face that clearly indicated silence.

"These walls have ears," Liu whispered. "Let us continue on to the temple to see my friend."

Liu started walking down the alley and stopped abruptly. Directly ahead, two men blocked the alley. Liu glanced back in the opposite direction and saw two more men slowly walking toward them. Liu knew instantly, by the way they walked and by their clothes, that these men were trained in some form of martial arts. After a few moves on their part, he would know their style, as well as what to watch out for. He needed to know where he would have the advantage. Each martial art had its strong point and its inherent weakness. That was the advantage to having studied many different styles.

In these close quarters, the expansive styles were at a disadvantage. Liu knew the fight would be unfair. Four against two, which actually was four against one, had to be over quickly. The four men would assume their numbers gave them the advantage, but in many such fights, unless the group coordinated the attack, they risked getting in each other's way, which would give Liu an advantage.

Pei Ke also saw the four men approaching and his stomach began to ache again. As he said "Master, are these the friends you are looking for?" he knew they were not.

"No, Pei Ke. These men are here to kill me. Unfortunately, you are here and they have decided your fate. Do exactly as I say."

He pulled a small double-edged knife from his robe and gave it to Pei Ke. Pei Ke was startled to see the knife emerge so quickly from somewhere in Liu's robe. Liu must have practiced this technique many times.

Pei Ke held the knife in his hand and wondered to which of the hundreds of gods he should pray. There must be some god to help in this situation. Maybe Kuan Yin will aid them.

He also wondered what exactly Master Liu expected him to do with the knife. Thankfully that question at least was quickly answered.

"Pei Ke, put your back against the wall. That will decrease the area you have to defend, and you will not have to worry about someone coming from behind. They will likely come for me rather than you. Your first instinct will be to stay close by for protection. It would be best for both of us if you stay close, but not too close. Move to the wall now."

"Yes, Master."

The four men closed in. One of the men spoke to Liu in a northern dialect. Liu replied in the same dialect.

Pei Ke did not know the dialect being spoken. He was surprised that this was the third dialect that Liu had spoken since starting their journey. He was close to dying, but he seemed unafraid of what might happen next.

Liu ignored the man who was speaking and instead watched the person closest to him. He had positioned himself in front of Pei Ke with two attackers on each side of him. He knew the attack would not come from the one closest to him, though he suspected Pei Ke thought so. It was a common ploy and Liu correctly assessed the situation.

The attack came from the heaviest of the four assailants. As soon as the attacker moved, Liu moved even faster to close the distance, catching the man off guard. He was only able to throw one punch towards Liu, but Liu was ready. He stepped to the left to block the punch, followed immediately with a Single Palm Change movement from Pa Kua Chang, which blocked the second punch, allowing him to move behind the attacker.

Receiving a flurry of sharp piercing jabs to the kidney and back area, the man fell to his knees in noticeable agony. The second assailant stepped forward closing the distance. With the Pi Chuan, a basic move from Hsing-Yi Chuan, Liu intercepted his punch. His follow through with the other hand landed on the assailant's collarbone and he was rewarded with the snapping of the assailant's collarbone and an agonizing cry. Liu raised his foot and kicked to the knee that was opposite the broken collarbone. The assailant immediately fell to the ground as Liu turned in the circling technique of Pa Kua Chang to face the other two.

Pei Ke watched Liu turn in circles to meet each one of the attackers, somehow managing to always be behind the attacker when the assault was launched. One by one, the attackers fell to the effects of various Pa Kua Chang, Hsing-Yi Chuan, and Tai Chi Chuan moves. The whole thing was over in less than fifteen seconds.

"Master…"

Pei Ke had to start again after catching his breath.

"Master, are they dead?"

"No. The first one is severely injured. He will never fight again. The second one has a broken collarbone—a difficult fracture to fix. He had a concealed knife and was about to draw it. I had no choice but to stop him. The other two are just unconscious. They will be able to tell their story when they return to whomever sent them."

"Master, you want them to return?"

"No, but I want them to worry about what they should do next. Doubt is always in my favor."

"Do we leave them here?" Pei Ke looked at the four men and wondered if they really knew what had happened.

"Yes, unless you want to stay here and befriend them."

Pei Ke handed the knife back to Liu and watched as it disappeared instantly into his robe. As they walked away from the area, Pei Ke looked back at the four men lying on the ground and felt proud to be in the company of such a powerful man.

"Who would want you dead, Master?" he said.

"That is what we are going to find out," Liu said. "Now, did you learn anything from that encounter?"

"That you are better than the stories told about you."

Again, despite his general disinterest in praise and acclaim, Liu was pleased by the company of his student. Pei Ke's enthusiasm, inquisitive nature and innocence were a welcome balance to the threat that was expressing itself more and more violently.

 "That is not an answer to my question."

"I'm sorry, Master. It seemed to me that you were always in control of the situation, no matter how they attacked or from which direction they came."

"What else did you learn?"

Pei Ke thought for a moment, unsure how to respond to his teacher. Was he looking for a compliment or did Master expect him to know every move he made?

"You were rooted to the ground and always knew what to do next."

"Once you have become proficient in martial arts, it is almost like a sixth sense. You are able to react and adjust to the slightest movement of your opponent. It takes years of practice, but it must be correct practice. If you practice the wrong movements all the time, you will fail when it comes time to defend yourself. Learn the applications and practice them by yourself, but you will never fully understand their dynamics if you do not practice the techniques with someone else. This applies to Tai Chi Chuan, Pa Kua Chang, and Hsing-Yi Chuan. Learning the forms of these arts without practicing the applications is useless."

They walked down one alley after another and Liu stopped often to ensure they were not being followed. Finally, they rounded a nondescript corner, and Pei Ke saw a small temple down a long, narrow, dead-end alley. As they drew near, they saw the interior of the temple. As with many temples, the entrance was the width of the building and opened into a main room with the altar at the back of the room and a life-size or larger statue behind the altar. Pei Ke did not recognize the image the statue represented. No one was in the temple. Pei Ke saw offerings on the floor and altar. Incense was burning in front of the altar.

Master Liu stopped and turned to his student.

"Pei Ke, my friend lives here with other monks in a semi-reclusive fashion. Do not ask questions or speak unless he asks you. If he speaks to you, address him as Master. He has no other name. The original name given to him by his father has been discarded as an earthly burden. You will see why shortly. Do you understand?"

"Yes, Master."

Liu motioned for Pei Ke to follow him. They walked around the right side of the temple to an old building in the back. Liu knocked on the door and, moments later, it slowly opened. The monk looked at Liu for a few seconds, smiled and nodded as he gestured for them to enter.

The inside was as spartan as the outside. Pei Ke saw a table and a few chairs and two doors leading somewhere.

Liu and the monk looked at each other without speaking. Pei Ke thought how eerie the atmosphere in the room had become. They just exchanged looks, sensing each other's energy. Finally, the monk turned to Pei Ke and bowed slightly. Pei Ke returned the greeting with a bow of deep respect.

The monk motioned for them to follow as he led them through one of the doors into a small room with a round table and chairs. Liu and the monk sat down, and Pei Ke followed their lead.

"Close your eyes and put your hands on the table," said the monk. Pei Ke did as instructed. He had an urge to open his eyes, but thought he better not. He needed to do as his master wanted.

"You two have come to me today," the monk said. "I sense a disruption in the universal energy. What affects the energy in one place is felt in another." He looked at Liu. "We have known each other for a long time. We both walk paths few others have taken. Your energy is strong. Stronger than most men. Your family's energy is part of you. When you move around the country, a part of that energy is always in constant touch with the other. That is how we sense things that we cannot explain. The energy is one, but it has numerous essences. As humans, we can tap into these various essences."

Pei Ke sensed that there was a sadness in his voice.

The monk stopped talking and Pei Ke felt the energy in his body shift. A connectedness between him and the monk was apparent. Pei Ke felt the monk entering into his own energy universe. It was both a strange feeling and a calming feeling. Pei Ke felt as if energy was moving through his body in search of a balance point. Just as quickly as it started, it stopped-and he felt a bliss he had not experienced before. He lost track of time and was startled when the monk spoke again.

"You both have come to see me to discover what lies ahead in your earthly journey. Since we are all inexplicably connected to the higher force of energy and your fortune will change as this energy changes, I can only tell you what will happen as it is set out for you now.

"Liu, you and I have entered into a world that few have traveled and few would want to travel. Each of us has given up a lot, but in return we have experienced more than anyone could ever hope for in this lifetime. I have experienced your energy as it relates to the overall universal energy, and I see many things that may appear to be contradictory. You will experience great danger and great sadness shortly. These will drive you to make decisions that violate tenets you hold dear to your heart. Your thirst for knowledge continues for some time and will take you afar. You will rise to higher levels of consciousness as you help others on the path to their higher levels. You will remain in good health for many years. One day you will be recognized for your great skills. Your immediate concern is with your family.

"Pei Ke, we have only met this one time. Your future is at a crossroads. Many roads will be opened to you shortly. You must choose which road to take. Fortunately, there are no wrong choices, only better choices. You will continue to search for Ancient Knowledge in ways you never expected. Affairs of the heart will come calling and you will need to address the implications of your actions.

"Liu, our paths have crossed more times than we can remember. I am still indebted to you for previous services. I trust I have been of some help to you today. It is time now for me to meditate. If you will excuse me. You are welcome to eat with us and stay the night."

The monk closed his eyes and his whole body relaxed. Without a word, Liu and Pei Ke rose from the table and walked out the door to the outer room and then into the alley.

"Pei Ke, do you believe what you just heard?"

"Master," Pei Ke said excitedly. "I felt this man's energy. It was unbelievable. He entered into my energy and it seems he now knows what I know, but I do not know any more than I did before." He sighed. "I'm sorry, Master, to answer your question, I believe what he told me is true but I do not know exactly what it means and I don't know what to do about it. Are there other people like him?"

"Many people learn esoteric skills. Each one of us is born with a unique ability. This ability comes from our parents and grandparents and is passed on to us. Because of everyone's uniqueness, many talents are possible. The fortunate ones like the monk realize their talents and cultivate them through training and study. Trying to force a talent is not always the right thing to do, especially if you do not have talent. If someone has a talent for medicine but no talent for martial arts, they will only have limited success if they try to be great at martial arts. It would be better for them to focus on medicine."

"Master, how do we know what is our specific talent?"

"I believe we are born with varying amounts of talents. For many who open themselves to the universal energy and go with the flow of energy, quite often they will discover an activity that is easy and enjoyable for them. That could well be their talent."

Liu and Pei Ke stayed and ate in silence with the monks as was the custom in the temple. Liu meditated most of the night as Pei Ke slept soundly. He barely even thought that his life had almost ended earlier. His experience with the monk seemed somehow more profound, more real, and it transformed the earlier violence into something more elegant and significantly less frightening, like a single element in a larger painting.

They rose early the next morning, practiced Qi Gong, and continued on their journey.

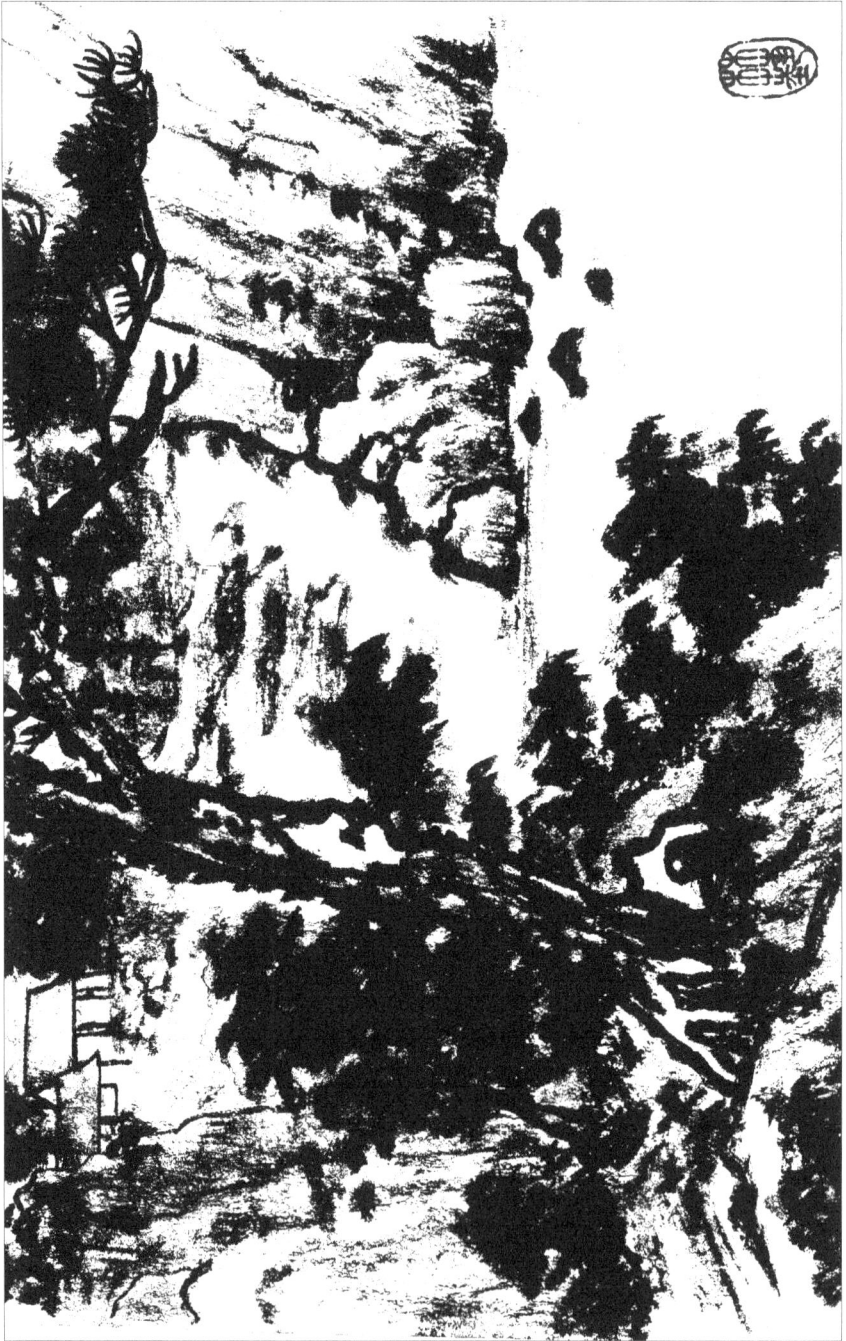

# CHAPTER FIFTEEN

Pei Ke, we must travel far today to keep on schedule. Let us walk faster for awhile. We will stop on the road ahead."

"Where are we stopping?"

"You will see when we get there."

Pei Ke hoped it was going to be a nice place. Maybe it was a special teahouse where they could get some tea and good food and perhaps take a little rest.

They walked in silence for a better part of the morning. Pei Ke walked with his knees slightly bent as Liu had instructed him to do that day. Each day, Liu changed either the way that Pei Ke walked or the manner in which Pei Ke held his hands or other parts of his body. He was sure he looked strange to those passing by. The looks from those passing by did not bother Liu.

Today Pei Ke had his palms facing down as if he were trying to make a connection with the center of the earth. He noticed a warm sensation in his palms and he could change the feeling by either moving his shoulders forward or backwards slightly. If he changed the position of his fingers a bit, he would get different sensations in his palms. He played with these various positions and combinations of shoulder, elbow, hand, wrist, and finger directions. He noticed Liu was watching out of the corner of his eye as this process continued.

"Have you found the perfect position yet?"

"I think so, Master. The more I experiment, the easier it is for me to identify when I have it correct. When it is correct, the feeling of Qi is balanced, and I have a sensation of being stronger. Plus, I feel wonderful sensations in my body."

"Yes. You are tapping into the universal energy. You are becoming both stronger and more rooted to the earth."

"Is there a physical limit to how much I can be rooted to the earth?" Pei Ke looked at the ground as he took the next few steps.

"Different techniques enhance this concept. Part of it is physical and part of it is mental. You must will it to happen. Train not only the body but also the mind if you want to be a good martial artist. The accomplished martial artists are able to root themselves so that they are virtually immovable."

"How do they do this?"

"Have you ever picked up a crying infant while it was twisting and turning?"

"Yes."

"You probably noticed it was more difficult to hold the infant and lift it up."

"Yes, I remember picking up little children and finding that when they wiggle, it is harder to control them."

Liu nodded. "When you can find the center of something, it is much easier to control that object or person. When it moves or wiggles, you must adjust your grip or body position to the motions to find the center."

The master occasionally gave Pei Ke a rest by allowing him to stand upright which would take the pressure off his legs and knees. Each time he straightened up he felt lighter and each time he resumed the bent walking position he felt more rooted to the earth. He thought to himself that this concept of rooting to the ground was both strange and exhilarating. He was becoming in a small way one with the earth.

Pei Ke knew Liu had thin but strong legs. Pei Ke's legs had become more sculptured from the constant practice of various walking exercises. Little or no fat existed on Pei Ke's body now, especially on his legs.

His shoulders also had more definition from the constant exercise. When he had been studying on the mountain, he would only practice two hours each day and then Liu would return to the temple. Now he was practicing all the time and he liked it. He could feel the discomfort in his body as he found new muscles he did not know he had, but he liked the feeling for it meant progress in his quest to be good in martial arts.

In addition to having more definition, his shoulder muscles were becoming rock hard from holding his hands in front of him with the palms facing upwards. When his hands faced downwards, he had one type of sensation and when his hands were facing upwards, he would have another type of sensation. He couldn't explain the different feelings. He had once seen Liu with his shirt off and remarked to Master how fit he was for someone his age. Liu had taken one of Pei Ke's fingers and placed it on top of his own shoulders. Liu extended his arms in the classic Pa Kua walking the circle posture and Pei Ke was amazed to feel a muscular indentation on top of the shoulder in the joint between the shoulder and the clavicle. Pei Ke was now developing this same muscular indentation in both of his own shoulders. He remembered Liu telling him that all Pa Kua practitioners have this telltale muscular indentation because of the training process.

"Pei Ke, we will leave the main road and follow this secondary road for a while. You must become familiar with an herb that grows here. It will only take us a few minutes. You may never get this chance again and it is important."

"Master, have you been this way before?"

"Yes, a friend of mine who is very knowledgeable about herbs took me here many years ago. We will not pick the herbs, but you need to see how they grow and what they look like. If you are ever asked, you can explain to your patient about the herb. The more knowledgeable you are, the more your patients will have confidence in your abilities."

They walked about ten minutes and Liu stopped to get his bearings. Then they continued on until Liu said "This is what we are looking for."

Pei Ke looked, but he could not distinguish one plant from another. He had only seen the herbs in the packages given to his parents, or in the large cabinet at the herbalist's shop. All he could remember was the taste of herbs. He knew each herb had its own unique qualities and he knew that herbs worked. Until now, that was all that had mattered to him, especially when he was so sick.

Liu pointed directly to a specific plant.

"This is Tang Kuei. Herbs have very specific properties. Some herbs dispel heat or cold and others balance the body. This herb has a number of different qualities. It relieves certain types of pain and can be combined with other herbs to accomplish specific objectives. It has another quality you need to remember. It tonifies and more specifically, it tonifies the blood. The *Divine Husbandman's Classic of the Materia Medica*, which was written in the second century, mentions this herb. It has been in use ever since.

"It has the properties of being sweet, acrid, and warm. Therapeutically it enters into the heart, spleen, and liver and tonifies the blood. It is one of the most important herbs in China for treating women's issues such as irregular menstruation, delayed periods, and painful periods. The herb when used after childbirth strengthens the blood of the mother. It is incredibly effective, but like all herbs there are contraindications and they should be used with caution."

"What are the contraindications with this herb? Is it safe to use?"

"Yes, it is safe to use when used appropriately. It is never used by itself, but rather in conjunction with other herbs based on the differential diagnosis of the patient and the patterns of disharmony existing in the patient's body. As an example, when this herb is prescribed you need to be careful the patient does not have diarrhea, since this herb has the tendency to lubricate the intestines. Therefore, in some instances, this herb when combined with other herbs can be used to treat symptoms of constipation."

"Master, why would it be helpful with women who have painful periods?"

"Painful periods can be due to a number of reasons. If the reason for the menstrual cramps is a blood deficiency condition in the uterus, then this herb can be used."

"Master, why can't just one herb be prescribed to solve these various women's issues?"

"I have explained this before. Each herb has a number of different properties. The differential diagnosis tells us the nature of the problem. Because of the properties of this specific herb, it is feasible to combine it with another herb that will counter the specific effects of causing the diarrhea."

Pei Ke thought for a moment. "So each herb has a number of different properties. Combinations of different herbs are used to specifically tailor the prescription for each individual patient with that specific problem at that specific time."

"Yes. Very good, that is correct," Liu said. "Doing otherwise may have an adverse effect. If you can remember to prescribe specifically for each patient, then your prescriptions will be effective. As you can guess, the key to the success of the herbal combination lies in your differential diagnosis. If your differential diagnosis is wrong, your prescription will be wrong. This applies not only to your herbal prescription, but also to your acupuncture prescription. You can't go into the shops and just buy one herb and expect it to work. In fact, it might do something entirely unexpected. So be careful."

"Yes, Master."

"Remember what this herb looks like in case you need to find it. The important part of the herb is the root. The herb is usually dug up and dried for later use. Next time we are in an herbalist's shop, we will look at different herbs that make up basic herbal formulas."

"Master, this is just one herb; how many different herbs do I need to remember?"

"There are hundreds of herbs you will eventually use in your lifetime, but you only need to remember about one hundred and fifty basic herbs. It takes time to learn, but if we take it slowly and consistently, you will remember not only the herb but how, why, and when to use them."

Liu turned and retraced his steps to the main road. Pei Ke took one last look at the Tang Kuei, turned, and followed Liu.

Pei Ke was deep in thought as they continued their journey north and after a brief time, Master Liu said, "Pei Ke. I know you have a question."

Pei Ke blushed, though he had not done so for many days now. Was he still so transparent?

"Master, you told me illness is basically an imbalance of the Qi, and we can solve this imbalance through acupuncture and herbs. Is one preferable over another? Which one is the best to use?"

"The imbalance in Qi can be solved through exercise like Tai Chi Chuan and Qi Gong, meditation, Tui Na, acupuncture, moxibustion, cupping, and herbs."

"Which one is the best?"

"They are all useful. The situation dictates which one is used. Internal problems of long duration can be solved with both acupuncture and herbs, but the herbs often work best when taken over time. Acupuncture works best for a pain problem of short duration. Cupping seems to work best with acute conditions when there is congestion like a cold, flu, and coughing. Gua Sha is appropriate when you want to disperse heat in the lungs. Gua Sha is appropriate for infants since they will not hold still for acupuncture. Moxibustion is good for chronic pain in the joints, especially if used in conjunction with acupuncture."

"Master, is there no end to these new words and ideas? What is Tui Na?"

Liu smiled.

"I will explain later. For now, just try to remember what I just told you."

"Yes, Master."

# Chapter Sixteen

On the eighth day, Liu and Pei Ke entered another province. They came to a small village with a crossroads. The road to Liu's parents' home went straight. At one time, the area was isolated, but as time went on, more and more people used the road to travel north and south.

The main street had wooden buildings lining both sides. Streets randomly branched off from the main road, much like an old gnarled tree. Each family wanted the front door facing a certain direction to conform to one or more specific birthdays. The local Feng Shui master had direct influence in the design of the village. Plots of land were seldom rectangular in design; rather, their design was based on the previous boundaries established by adjacent owners and the need to conform to Feng Shui for the next resident of the adjacent property.

As was typical of small villages in remote areas, everyone knew everyone else, therefore, a new face always brought suspicion. The local villagers had a tendency to stare at strangers, and Pei Ke was uncomfortably aware of the stares as they walked down the dusty street.

"Master, have you ever been through this village before? Do you know anyone in this village?"

"I have been this way before, but I have never stopped in the village."

Pei Ke moved closer to Liu. He straightened his shoulders and tightened his grip on his sack.

"Master, there is something strange about this village. The way people are staring is different from the looks we've received in other villages. I feel something sinister or evil is here."

Liu thought it was interesting that Pei Ke felt that way. The last time he had traveled through here he had the same feeling. Maybe his father's stories about this area were true. Previously, Liu had only half believed those stories, but now he found the coincidence was too great to discount.

"Pei Ke, have you ever walked into a room of people and felt uncomfortable, or been approached by someone and felt uncomfortable?"

"Yes, and that is how I feel about this place, but even more so. It's almost cold. It is quite different from other villages we've passed through."

"Some places have an accumulation of energy. In most instances, this energy is favorable. In other words, it affects people in a good way. People identify with the place and usually remark that they feel comfortable there. Many times, that place is in the mountains or by the seaside, or is close to a natural phenomenon like a waterfall, or a geyser, or a mature forest.

"But other places have the opposite effect. Luckily, these are few. Both you and I feel it in this place. Others who have passed through here probably felt it. My father felt it whenever he was here. Maybe the energy of the land or the energy of the villagers is not good. Perhaps the Feng Shui master was inept and the buildings and the development of the land are wrong."

"Master, could it be evil spirits lurking in the area? My parents told me about such things and I remember as a child being afraid of the spirits. I wondered where they lived. Maybe this is the place." Despite his sudden discomfort at the thought of evil spirits, he was happy to know that the master felt the same discomfort about the place.

"If you believe in evil spirits," the master said, "it is possible that belief is what gives us this feeling. The evilness of the world can spread out and affect those passing through its area of influence. It is almost like the concept of evil Qi in medicine. Evil Qi can attack the healthy body. If the body is not strong, the evil Qi will overcome the good Qi and cause disease. The evil Qi invades from the external and penetrates to the internal. Maybe this is what has happened to this village."

Liu and Pei Ke continued to walk into the village area. They saw the usual sights and sounds of vendors selling their wares and shops selling delicacies to eat. As they walked, it seemed as if those who walked towards them went out of their way to avoid them. They both noticed that the temperature dropped as they got closer and closer to the center of the village.

"Master, I know we are walking north and the temperature should be getting cooler, but there is a coolness or coldness in the earth which seems to enter my feet and move up my legs."

"I have felt it also."

"Master, are we going to stay here long? Maybe we should move on quickly before the evil spirits find out we are passing through their territory. Maybe they don't like us trespassing."

Liu slowed his pace. "I have always passed through, but I think we should stay for a while. Usually a village of this size has a temple. We have walked for a long time and we are both thirsty and hungry. People at the temple may be kind enough to give us some water and food."

"Master," Pei Ke said with a boldness he usually reserved for asking questions. "I am thirsty and hungry. I have never questioned anything you have done, but this place makes me uncomfortable. Please, can we leave soon and find food and water somewhere else?"

"Perhaps, follow me."

Liu knew temples were usually located in auspicious locations to appease the various gods. Like everything else, Feng Shui dictated the location and design. Liu looked at the surrounding hillsides and noticed a building resembling a Buddhist temple and started toward it. Pei Ke hesitantly followed. At first, Pei Ke began to fall behind, but as the distance between them increased, a feeling of apprehension and then terror engulfed Pei Ke. He quickly ran to catch up.

The twists and bends of the streets were deceptive and despite their efforts, they could not seem to find their way to the temple. Somehow, they always returned to the main street and the temple peeked at them to their right. Finally, as they approached the edge of the village, Pei Ke saw a sign, but he did not say anything. He hoped Liu did not see it.

"Pei Ke, the sign indicates that the temple is down this little path. It is the Temple of the Living Swallow. A strange name for a temple, which I presume is a Buddhist temple. Follow me."

"Master, maybe I will wait for you here."

"Pei Ke, if you stay here I cannot protect you from those evil spirits. It is better to be with me than to be on your own."

Pei Ke thought for a moment and ran to catch up with the master, who again walked at a brisk pace. The road led uphill but Liu did not slow down. In fact, he picked up the pace, which made Pei Ke run even faster to catch up with him.

As Liu was walking, he took in all that was around him. He noticed the land and crops did not look healthy. Their growth was stunted, almost as if the growing process had been interrupted before the crops came to maturity. The bamboo in the distance should be tall instead of growing sideways. The place was depressing. Something was wrong here. Liu wondered if Pei Ke had been right and that they should leave and do without food and water.

Liu turned quickly at the first sound of Pei Ke's scream. Two men were pulling the sack from Pei Ke, and he was struggling to hold on with both hands. He had no chance to defend himself. Liu covered the distance swiftly.

One of the men let go of the sack, took out a throwing star and with a quick flick of his arm and wrist sent the star toward Liu. As the star approached his heart, the master instinctively stepped to the side and turned his waist to decrease the surface area under attack. The star grazed his clothes but did not scratch his skin. Liu knew it was likely poisoned and without breaking stride, he continued toward Pei Ke before another star was thrown.

Out of the corner of his eye, Liu saw two more men rising from the bushes by the road ready to join in the fight. He knew he would not have a second chance. Unless he dispatched each one of them on first contact, he would not survive this encounter and neither would Pei Ke. There were just too many of them and this time, they had as much room as they wanted. They would not attack him in turns. They would gang up. Briefly he wondered if Pei Ke would find a way to help, or if he would be the handicap that would spell their end.

Pei Ke did not see the whole fight; he was too busy protecting the sack Liu had entrusted to him. He did hear an agonizing scream and the sound of a bone breaking, followed by a crunching sound, and a deep exhalation of air. The man grabbing the sack released his grip. Pei Ke watched him and the last man standing run down the hill. Two men lay dead on the ground next to their knives. One man's head was twisted in an abnormal way and blood ran from the other man's mouth. Liu had a small scratch on his wrist. Pei Ke looked at Liu and could see that he was solemn and deep in thought.

"Master, why did they attack us?"

Liu did not answer. Instead he bent down and looked closely at the faces of the men who had attacked them. Pei Ke could see a sincere and overpowering sadness in Liu's face. He knelt down next to one of the men and leaned over until he was inches from the man's face. Liu sniffed, then rose. He was about to speak to Pei Ke when they felt a coldness descend from the upper part of the road. They looked toward the temple and saw a distant figure turn and walk back inside the building.

"Why did they attack us?" Pei Ke said again. "We are peaceful travelers passing through. We mean no harm to anyone."

"Evilness takes many forms," Liu said. "Sometimes the evilness is inside a person at birth. Sometimes a person's evilness is due to the evilness of another person. This place is evil because of the evilness of people who are extending their influence on others."

He rose to his feet and gestured to the body on the road.

"This man was an addict. He was forced by someone else to do evil in exchange for drugs. People who prey on others are the scourge of the earth. They don't contribute anything to society and only cause the breakdown of the moral structure of both the individual and the surrounding society. These men were after whatever any travelers had of value.

"Travelers have no choice but to continue on their way, even if they lose their belongings. The robbers know no one will listen to complaints since it appears everyone in the area is under the influence of this evilness. I hold no animosity toward these men. They are controlled by another. This is a good lesson for you to remember in your journeys throughout life. In instances where situations do not seem right to you, do what your conscience tells you. If there is any wavering about good and evil, avoid the circumstances that would put you in harm's way."

"Master, these men are dead. Will the authorities want to question us about their death?"

"I don't think so. It is unlikely that anyone has governmental authority here in this village. It is probably run by a local magistrate who ignores controversy."

"Should we bury the bodies, or take them somewhere for others to look after?"

"No, leave them where they fell."

Liu looked at the temple one last time and retraced his steps down the side road to the main road that would take him to his brother's house. Pei Ke stayed alongside him, constantly looking in different directions. When they got to the northern outskirts of the village, the coldness of the weather and the coldness of the evilness gradually dissipated. By then neither man felt thirsty nor hungry. They had another three hours before they would rest for the evening. As they walked, each was deep in thought. Liu was thinking about his family, wondering what evil had befallen them, and was anxious to make up lost time. He did not like to kill and he hoped that in any future conflict that lay before him, he would not have to kill again. The words of the monk clung to him like smoke and the day's mêlée had done nothing to reassure him.

Pei Ke's thoughts were not so personal, but were nearly as weighty. He simply contemplated good and evil, and wondered how often goodness won out over evilness.

# CHAPTER SEVENTEEN

On the ninth day, they awoke early and quickly continued on their journey. Pei Ke's legs and lungs soon told him they were climbing to higher and higher elevations as they headed north.

"Pei Ke, we need to walk a little faster; we have a long way to go today before we rest for the night."

"Master, where will we be staying?"

"At a unique place. One of my students has a clinic in the mountains. It is associated with an adjacent temple. He has dedicated his life to helping others who are less fortunate. He accepts only donations for his treatments. If he gets too many donations, he uses the excess to improve the clinic or he gives the money to the monks. He started the clinic when his wife passed away at an early age. Whenever I am traveling on this road, I visit him for at least one night.

"He is a good doctor and he knows some martial arts. He is in tune with the universal healing energy in ways most doctors can only dream about. He originally came to me to study martial arts but soon realized his true passion was medicine. You can learn a lot from him. He also has a unique ability with Feng Shui."

Throughout the journey Pei Ke could see the changing landscape. The more they spent time in the mountains the better he felt. He didn't know if it was the trees or the higher elevations, but he liked it.

"Master, does your friend make contact with the spirits?"

"No, I don't think so. He was born with a gift to see energy, auras, and colors of different energy. We all are born with this gift. The majority of us, however, lose the gift as we age. He was fortunate to retain his. He uses the gifts given to him rather than hide the gifts. He is also a very good diagnostician. His acupuncture prescriptions and herbal prescriptions have helped many people. His ability is based on years of experience and study."

They walked for much of the day with Liu answering questions and Pei Ke developing strength and stamina from doing the moves of Pa Kua Chang and Hsing-Yi Chuan. As they climbed, the trees turned from broadleaf trees to scattered pine trees, to dense pine forests.

"It is only a couple more miles," Liu said. "The uphill climb will help develop your legs."

"If I had any fat it would surely be burnt off during this walk," puffed Pei Ke.

Liu smiled to himself. The boy would not have lasted through the abusive training regime he had endured.

The sign "Tsao's Clinic" was written in big red characters. Liu and Pei Ke took the side road indicated on the sign and walked for a quarter mile up an even steeper incline. As they walked, the forest on both sides of the path became denser. Pei Ke breathed in the smell of pine trees.

"Sick people could never climb this road," thought Pei Ke. "If they could make it up the road to the clinic, they must not be too sick."

They had walked less than a mile when Pei Ke heard a faint sound in the distance. As they continued along the road, the sound increased in intensity.

Pei Ke asked. "Master, what is that sound?"

"It is a waterfall. You will see shortly."

Pei Ke had never heard the roar of cascading water. It sounded ominous like the power of a spring storm. His curiosity was answered as they reached the source of the noise. Pei Ke saw a large waterfall with a walking bridge connecting the two sides. He stopped for a second to catch the beauty of what was before him. The whole scene reminded him of one of the paintings he had seen back at the teahouse. With Liu in the lead, they walked across the swaying foot bridge. He could feel the mist coming off the churning water. As he looked down, he felt slightly dizzy. He grabbed hold of the ropes to regain his balance. He held on to the ropes as he continued across to the opposite side. When they walked off the bridge, Pei Ke turned around to once again see the beauty of the waterfall. Liu walked up the incline leading away from the bridge without saying a word.

At the top of the incline, the ground leveled off and Pei Ke saw the temple and the nearby clinic. A scattering of houses surrounded the temple. Fruit trees and gardens filled much of the remaining area, making it look beautiful and tranquil. The peacefulness of the landscape appealed to Pei Ke. He thought he could live here for the rest of his life.

They walked through the grounds toward the main clinic area. Word of their arrival must have preceded them as Dr. Tsao appeared in the front doorway, waiting for them.

He was short, with well kept clothes and appearance, as one might expect a doctor to look. Tsao's appearance stood out in contrast to Liu, who was clean-looking, but whose appearance gave no impression of his medical expertise.

"Master, again welcome to my humble clinic," Tsao Cheng said.

"Cheng, this is Pei Ke. He is traveling with me on the way home. Do you have room for us for the night?"

"Of course. There is always room for you. In fact, I am still waiting for you to accept my offer to stay here permanently and help me with the patients."

"Perhaps someday I will accept your gracious offer, but for now we need only to stay the night. We will be on our way early in the morning. We hope not to disturb you in your work."

"You are tired and probably need to rest. Let me show you to your rooms."

"We are not tired," said Liu.

Pei Ke barely kept himself from complaining. Exhaustion permeated his body from the day's march and the grand climb to the clinic had drained him even more. Master Liu would run both of them into the ground.

"I was just visiting with my patients when you arrived. Would you like to come with me?"

"Of course," Liu said.

Without looking at Pei Ke, Liu, and the doctor entered the clinic.

"Master, where should I put the sack?"

"Hold on to it and follow."

The three of them walked down the hallway to the first ward where some male patients were laying on beds. Staff members and patients were in the hallway and all paid respect to the three of them. For Pei Ke, it was a new experience. He liked the idea of being treated like an important person.

"Cheng, is it all right for Pei Ke to accompany us? I have accepted him as a student. He is interested in medicine and one day wants to be a doctor."

"Of course. Pei Ke, you are most welcome. I remember the first day I studied from Master Liu. I had no idea what to expect. Everyone said it was such a great honor. Even to this day, it is an honor when he comes to visit.

"While we are walking, I will tell you about my clinic. Perhaps it can be of some use to you on your own path. When I studied with Master Liu, I would feel so good when I saw the results of the healing process. I decided I wanted to do something special for humanity. Maybe it was my addiction to feeling good about myself when my patients got well. I can't really explain the feeling except to say it was like a mental euphoria. The more the patients improved, the more euphoric I became, and the more I wanted the patients to get well. I found some things in life that mattered more than wealth and material possessions.

"This profession could easily make me rich like so many of my colleagues. It would be easy to have a summer home like the Emperor and travel to various places, but I realized those are only external fulfillments and not a means to internal happiness. Let them have their accumulated things of wealth. I have what counts inside. This is due in part, of course, to our master and his teachings and philosophy. The more I give the more I receive in return.

"Here in the clinic we treat a wide range of health related issues. We will accept anyone with a problem; however, we are known best for taking in patients who have problems not readily solved by other means: bursitis, insomnia, constipation, diarrhea, low back and hip pain, knee pain, sciatica, neuropathy, carpal tunnel syndrome, and internal problems."

They walked into the men's ward. The ward was a large room with all of its fifteen beds filled with patients. Doctors were treating the patients with acupuncture, moxibustion, and Tui Na. The wonderful sense of peacefulness in the ward was similar to the peacefulness Pei Ke had experienced when he had first seen the buildings and the surrounding landscape.

"Master Liu and some of my other teachers were kind enough to share their accumulated learning with me," Cheng said. "Now I share my knowledge with others. Ten doctors are in training here. The teaching method follows the ancient tradition, exactly how Master taught me.

"We discuss each patient and then I give the doctors a discourse on the patient's problem and they watch how I treat that problem. The doctors experience a continual hands-on approach from the first day they enter training. In addition to my teaching, their education is supplemented with their own readings. Contact with actual patients is necessary for the doctors to learn. In essence, each patient is both a lecture and practical experience.

"This teaching method is different from what is taught at other schools or hospitals. In many places the students spend two to three years learning basic knowledge with no practical experience. At the end of book learning and lecture phase of the training, there is a period of limited clinical experience. I personally think these young students are being shortchanged."

"Doctor Tsao, where do these patients come from?" asked Pei Ke.

"Mainly from within fifty miles of the clinic. Other doctors refer some of their patients to us. Some are referred by other temples in the area whose monks are aware of the clinic. Quite often, patients hear about us through word of mouth. Regardless of how they hear of us, we turn no one away. If they have money they make a donation. If they have no money, they can pray for the success of the clinic. Either way, the universal energy will look favorably on this place of healing."

"How many students or doctors do you have here?"

"It varies from time to time, but right now there are two other doctors besides myself and ten students in training."

"What are your criteria for the students you accept?"

"I require someone to visit with me and explain in detail why he or she wants to be a doctor. When I tell them it will take at least four years and they don't get paid, it usually eliminates a good percentage of the potential students."

Doctor Tsao took Liu and Pei Ke around to meet the doctors and students. Liu recognized one of the doctors from a previous visit. They all knew who Liu was and paid the utmost respect to him.

"Master, are you sure you are up for making some rounds with me? I could use some of your advice on the more difficult cases."

"Yes, we are both ready," said Liu. "Lead the way."

Doctor Tsao stopped at one bed and introduced Liu and Pei Ke to the patient. Tsao turned to the patient and asked permission to discuss the problem with his teacher. The patient agreed.

"Master, this patient complains of a persistent cough. He indicates the coughing has been continuous for about one week. In addition to the coughing, he has a scratchy throat, headache, stuffy nose, and a fever. When we checked his tongue, it had a white coating. His pulses are weak and superficial. We have done a thorough differential diagnosis and have determined his problem is due to an external invasion of a pathogenic factor. Specifically, we feel, since the weather is turning colder and the wind is blowing harder, he has a wind cold syndrome. He came in yesterday and we will treat him for a few days."

Liu felt the patient's pulses and looked at his tongue.

"Your diagnosis appears to be correct," Liu said. "What acupuncture and herbal prescription are you using?"

Tsao explained the acupuncture points used and the herbal formulation given to the patient.

"Your diagnosis is correct and the prescriptions are good. He should be better within two to three days with no complications. In these situations, we are concerned about the pathogenic factors going deeper into the lungs and causing further damage. Your prescription will prevent that from happening and help with a rapid recovery."

With the second patient, Tsao related the patient's problem and the method of treatment. Liu felt the pulses and looked at the patient's tongue. Tsao Cheng explained the herbal formulation and acupuncture points being used.

"This patient, like the first, has a lung problem, but the problem is totally different in nature," Liu said. "Yes, he coughs a little but the problem is not from an external pathogenic factor. As you correctly ascertained, giving him the same acupuncture and herbal prescriptions as the first patient would be of little benefit. Your prescriptions for him are good. You might want to have him do Qi Gong in the early morning in the nearby forests. The pine trees will help him especially if he does deep breathing. At first it may be a little difficult for him, but he should see some quick results."

"Doctor Tsao, may I ask a question?" Pei Ke said timidly.

Tsao turned to Pei Ke and looked at him for an extended period of time, which made Pei Ke uncomfortable Tsao said "Yes, you may ask."

"We have seen two patients with a cough and they are being treated differently. How many different cough patterns are there?"

"Coughing can be differentiated into maybe ten to fifteen different patterns, all treated differently with acupuncture and herbal formulations. These patterns are either internal or external. The internal can be further divided by excess or deficiency."

Doctor Tsao appeared to be very good at what he did. Pei Ke wondered if maybe he was better than Master Liu.

Liu went to the third patient. Doctor Tsao talked with the patient for a few minutes and then turned to Liu.

"Master, this patient has arthritis in both knees and in his back and neck. He has had the problem for two to three years, and it is getting progressively worse. The problem first started in his knees, then went to his lower back, and now is in his neck. He thinks his arthritis will move to his shoulders and hands next. He is in quite a bit of pain. His arms and legs feel heavy and his ankles are swollen. His tongue, when he arrived a week ago, was a normal color, but had a white greasy fur on the surface."

"What type of work do you do?" Liu asked the man.

The patient rubbed his hands over his face. "I am from the valley area. We have rice fields. Actually, I need to be there now working, but the pain is so bad there is little I can do. I am more of a hindrance than a help. Do you know why I have such pain?" He leaned back on his elbows to rest his back.

"How old are you? How long have you been a rice farmer?' Liu asked.

"I am fifty-two years old and have been working in the fields since I was a child."

"Pei Ke."

"Yes, Master."

"This type of problem happens sometimes to people who work with water up to their knees. It is probably a dampness problem. Doctor Tsao, how are you treating the problem?"

"We came to the same conclusion as you did, and we are trying to lessen the dampness. Local acupuncture therapy and heat therapy are helping."

Liu turned to the patient. "How have you been since starting the treatments?"

"When I came in a couple of weeks ago, I could barely walk. It physically hurt and I was tired. It still hurts, but it is much better now. I am seeing daily improvement with the treatments. Doctor Tsao is really an excellent doctor. He is a very kind man."

For the next two hours Liu, Tsao and Pei Ke made the rounds from one patient to another. Sometimes Liu would make recommendations and sometimes he would only nod his head in agreement. Pei Ke found the process stimulating but tiring. He had walked all day and was at the point of exhaustion.

He was both disappointed and relieved when Tsao said, "Master, that is our last patient for tonight. There are more for tomorrow, if you want to see them."

"I would like to see all the patients," Master Liu said, "but we need to be on our way at first light tomorrow morning." Pei Ke noticed that as he said this, a heaviness came into his voice. He looked at Tsao and was sure the doctor had noticed it too.

# CHAPTER EIGHTEEN

During their journey, Liu continued to instruct Pei Ke in martial arts, medicine, and philosophy. As they walked, Liu had Pei Ke hold his arms in various outstretched positions. These Hsing-Yi Chuan and Pa Kua Chang positions developed upper body strength. The crouched walking positions of Hsing-Yi Chuan and Pa Kua Chang developed lower body strength. He watched intently as his student grew physically stronger day by day.

As they walked, Liu answered all questions Pei Ke asked. He knew that the boy's concentration on his questions and answers Liu provided would divert Pei Ke's mind from the pain he was experiencing, but it also helped divert Liu's mind from what he knew lay ahead.

On the eleventh day, he estimated that they were slightly ahead of schedule and would be at his father's house sooner than he had expected. Still, he picked up the pace just a little.

"Master, I have been holding my arms in this Pa Kua Chang position for over half an hour. My arms and shoulders are beginning to ache."

"Master Tung Hai Chuan would maintain this posture for much longer than this while walking the circle. He would have a cup in the palm of each hand filled to the brim with water. The goal was to walk the circle for an extended period of time and not spill any of the water. You are not walking in circles, but you will get the benefit just the same. If you are too tired, you can put your arms down."

Pei Ke continued to keep his arms extended in front and to the side. He imagined there was a cup of water in each hand and he was not going to let the water spill.

"There are numerous books on classical Chinese Medicine. I have mentioned some of them to you and have shared with you information from quite a few. One of the first and most important is the *Yellow Emperor's Classic of Internal Medicine* written by Huang Ti. If you can remember, understand thoroughly, and apply all that is in this book, you will be a superior doctor.

"Huang Ti mentions that doctors fail in their care of patients in a number of different ways. You need to understand these failings so you will become a better doctor." He noticed the quivering in Pei Ke's arms. "If your arms are getting tired you can put them down and rest for a few minutes."

"I'm alright."

"The first failing is an improper or wrong diagnosis. This happens when doctors do not take enough time to ascertain the true problem of the patient. It is not possible to spend one to two minutes with a patient and then write an herbal prescription or a prescription for acupuncture.

It is also important to analyze the emotional state of the patient. Quite often, the emotional state of the patient may affect the energy system of the body. In addition, a doctor should learn where the patient fits within the individual's social structure. Quite often social activities cause stress and stress impacts the energy system.

"The second failing is also quite common. It is where a treatment is being performed without a complete understanding of the concept of tonification and dispersion. If tonification is applied when dispersion is needed, the patient will probably get worse. The same with dispersion. If dispersion is applied where tonification is needed, the patient will probably get worse.

"The third failing is the lack of understanding about the four diagnostic procedures. This is because the doctor does not have a full grasp of the concepts of Yin and Yang and the theory of Five Elements.

"The fourth failing occurs when the doctor does not provide the patient enough information about their particular condition and how to resolve it.

Sometimes all a patient needs is some guidance as to why something has happened to him. The patient relies on the doctor to help him overcome the health care issues. Do everything you can to help your patient understand what is happening.

"The fifth failing of a doctor is his lack of concern, which may lead to negligence. It is important to remember to do the patient no harm. The patient has trusted you with his health concerns. Do justice to that relationship, and do not violate the confidence and trust placed in you as a doctor.

"These are the words of Huang Ti written over a thousand years ago. They are still true today, but to these five failings, I am going to add two more.

"The sixth failing is to discount what a patient tells you is a symptom. What the patient feels—whether it is physical, emotional, or psychological—is real to him. He is experiencing it firsthand. Who are you to tell the patient it is not real? If the patient tells you he has sore areas on a number of locations on his body and the pain is getting worse over time, it does not make sense to give them herbs to relax his mind, and then give him stronger and stronger herbs to totally sedate him when the problem does not exist in his mind. The problem is multifaceted and it is your responsibility to discover the complexity of the energy imbalance and not mask it.

"The seventh and final failing concerns prescribing herbal formulas or giving acupuncture treatments. The body can only make so many adjustments. Don't overload the patient. It is always your responsibility to make sure you know the interactions of all the herbs you are prescribing and to ascertain from the patient what other herbs they are taking."

Pei Ke felt a heavy burden placed on his shoulders.

"Do you have any questions?"

"No, Master. Being a doctor sounds like a tremendous responsibility."

"Yes. Unfortunately many doctors do not take enough time to do a complete evaluation on the patient. Pei Ke!"

"Yes, Master?"

"Put your arms down."

Pei Ke had forgotten that his arms had been in that strange position for such a long time. The pain dissipated as he lowered his arms. The two walked past several fields. Pei Ke shook his arms and wiggled his fingers.

Liu stopped and faced Pei Ke. "Now I would like you to place your hands next to your body, your elbows slightly bent and your palms facing downwards towards the ground. What do you feel?"

Pei Ke did as Liu said. He had done this movement so many times before that he knew exactly how Liu wanted it done.

"Master, as usual, I can feel the energy in my body, but today it seems to be more intense than before."

"Good! You are making progress. Your joints are opening more so the energy can flow more freely than before. Now bend your legs just a little bit more."

Pei Ke again did as instructed. He had walked with his legs slightly bent ever since he met Liu. At first, the pain was intense, but he gradually got use to it and had learned to ignore it. He was definitely getting stronger. With this intense daily regimen of exercise, he was making progress much faster than he had ever done before.

# Chapter Nineteen

)n the early afternoon of the twelfth day of traveling, Liu and Pei Ke entered a small community. Those passing by nodded in greeting as Liu and Pei Ke casually strolled down the dirt streets.

"Master, where are we staying tonight?"

"I do not know. I don't know anyone in this area. It may be too late in the afternoon to make it to the next community. I do not want to sleep out in the open, unless I need to. The universal energy will provide for what is best."

Liu saw an elderly couple walking towards them. As they approached, he stopped. "Excuse me. We are travelers in need of food and a place to stay for the night. Do you know if we could find work in exchange for food and lodging?"

The old couple shook their head and walked on. Liu approached five other individuals and posed the same question. Each one responded similarly. Everyone seemed friendly, but no one wanted to take a chance with travelers. Pei Ke had mixed feelings about having to beg for food and lodging. He had never begged for anything prior to this journey. He was always poor, but never to the point where he had no food.

"Master, you are a great person. Why do you have to beg for food and lodging?"

"The higher one's station in life, the more onerous it is to ask for food. In this situation it is not begging for food. It is a willingness to exchange my talents for food and lodging. The accumulation of material things or the want of material things causes us to feel superior. When you think about people, no matter who we are and what station in life we have been assigned, no one person is any greater than another. Is the life of a child from a poor family any different than a life of a child from a rich family?"

"Master, I know we are all human beings, but there is something degrading about having no money, and it seems even more degrading about having to beg for food and a place to stay."

Liu talked with more people as the day wore on and finally, someone indicated there was a house a couple of streets up where one might find some work and a place to stay for the night. Liu and Pei Ke walked up the street and knocked on the door of the house. The door opened, they saw a woman in her mid-forties holding a small child. Laughter coming from somewhere in the house indicated that there were other children at play.

Liu introduced himself. "We are traveling north and are in need of food and shelter. A kind individual on the street mentioned that you may be able to help us. We are willing to work this evening for your help."

"Where are you from?" the woman asked.

"I reside at a temple to the south of here. Pei Ke is one of my students and is traveling with me."

"If he is your student, what do you teach?"

"Pei Ke is studying martial arts and medicine from me."

"I need some wood chopped."

"Pei Ke will be happy to do that for you. Just show him what to do."

"What can you do?"

"What do you need done?"

"I need some water hauled from the well to the kitchen."

"Pei Ke can do that for you as well. Do you have any health problems needing attention? I am experienced with acupuncture and herbal formulas."

"Come in. You can sleep in the extra room at the back of the house. Give me a few minutes and I will bring you some food. After you finish eating, then you can help me. You can put your things in the back room now."

After eating, Pei Ke chopped the wood as instructed and hauled water from the community well to the kitchen barrel. While Pei Ke was doing his chores, Liu attended to the woman.

After finishing the chores, Pei Ke sat down with Liu in the back room.

"I don't know why I had to chop the wood and haul the water. She had plenty of wood already chopped and the water barrel had at least two days worth of water."

"It was her way of exchanging value for value," said Liu. "She told me her husband died two years ago from a mysterious disease. She is raising her four children by herself on this small piece of land. The neighbors help a little, but she does rely on strangers sometimes to do some odd jobs for her. At the moment, she does not have any odd jobs, but she always needs wood chopped for the stove. Helping another person almost always gives me a warm feeling. Some people have a difficult life. My life is by my own choosing, but others are not as fortunate. They have a burden whether situational or because of their past lives."

"Master, may I ask some questions?"

"Yes."

"What is wrong with this kind woman?"

"She had pain in both of her hips, legs, and feet. As I have told you before, our health care issues are due to an imbalance in the energy flow in our bodies. This imbalance can be due to a number of different factors. The imbalance can be due to a structural problem. It can be due to lifestyle. It can be due to injuries she has sustained. It can be due to the weather. It can be due to emotions. For her, after going through the diagnostic process, I suspect that her problem is due to a previous injury to her lower back. She is constantly lifting her young children, which may aggravate the problem. She felt much better after the treatment."

"Master."

"Yes."

"Before my father passed away, he suffered pain and numbness in his legs and feet. Could acupuncture have helped him?"

"That is a broad question. I can only go by what you tell me. What were his symptoms?"

"As he got older he started to get tingling and numbness in his toes. It got worse over the course of a year when it started to spread to his feet and legs. He complained that his legs and feet hurt. The bottom of his feet felt like cotton. Even though he felt a lot of pain, the numbness and loss of feeling caused him to lose balance. After awhile, walking became difficult. Based on what I just told you, could you have helped him?"

"Of course a differential diagnosis is essential. However, in general these types of problems usually respond well to acupuncture treatments. I have treated many very successfully."

"What could cause the problem?"

"It could be related to diabetes, with diminished circulation to the extremities. It could be lower back problems or some other condition where there is an imbalance or blockage of energy flow. It usually affects older people. It can be quite debilitating. A diabetic patient can actually lose a leg because of severe lack of circulation. Quite often, the patient will start to receive relief after a few visits. Of course if treatment had started at the early stages of the problem, there is a greater probability of success than if treatment is started years after the problem has begun."

"Master may I ask you some questions about martial arts?"

"Yes."

"You know your family's martial arts plus the internal martial arts. What else do you know?"

"The three internal martial arts are similar in many ways and there has been cross training in all three. Even so, when you train in each of these, each has unique characteristics that make it easy to switch from one to another. Usually, but not always, a practitioner will be better in one of the three.

"When the arts are too dissimilar, the underlying principles are too divergent and the arts do not easily mesh together. Because Tai Chi Chuan, Pa Kua Chang, and Hsing-Yi Chuan have some commonality, it is possible to switch from one to another with relative ease.

"To answer your question, I also know Chin Na, Fa Jing, sword, double sword, broad sword, deer horn knives, staff, and other weapons. Right now, Chin Na is the most important aspect of your training. Chin Na refers to the use of joint locks, pressure points, and muscle separation in martial arts to subdue an opponent. I have already shown you some of these moves."

"Master, could you show me some more?"

"The art of Chin Na is effective in controlling your opponent. Pei Ke, with your right hand I want you to grasp my right wrist."

Pei Ke grasped Liu's right wrist. Liu's left hand came down on top of Pei Ke's right hand trapping the hand. There was a slight pull forward and an instant later, with virtually no force Pei Ke felt an intense pain in his wrist running up his arm to his shoulder. The pain was so intense and the leverage against his wrist joint so pronounced that Pei Ke dropped to his knees. Liu immediately released the grip, not wanting to follow through with the rest of the technique which would have caused severe injury to Pei Ke.

"Stand up," he said to Pei Ke, who was still kneeling on the floor. "I will show you more."

For the next hour, Liu showed Pei Ke numerous Chin Na techniques used against various grabs and punches. At the end of the hour, Pei Ke was both sore and exhilarated. He had learned a lot in a short period of time.

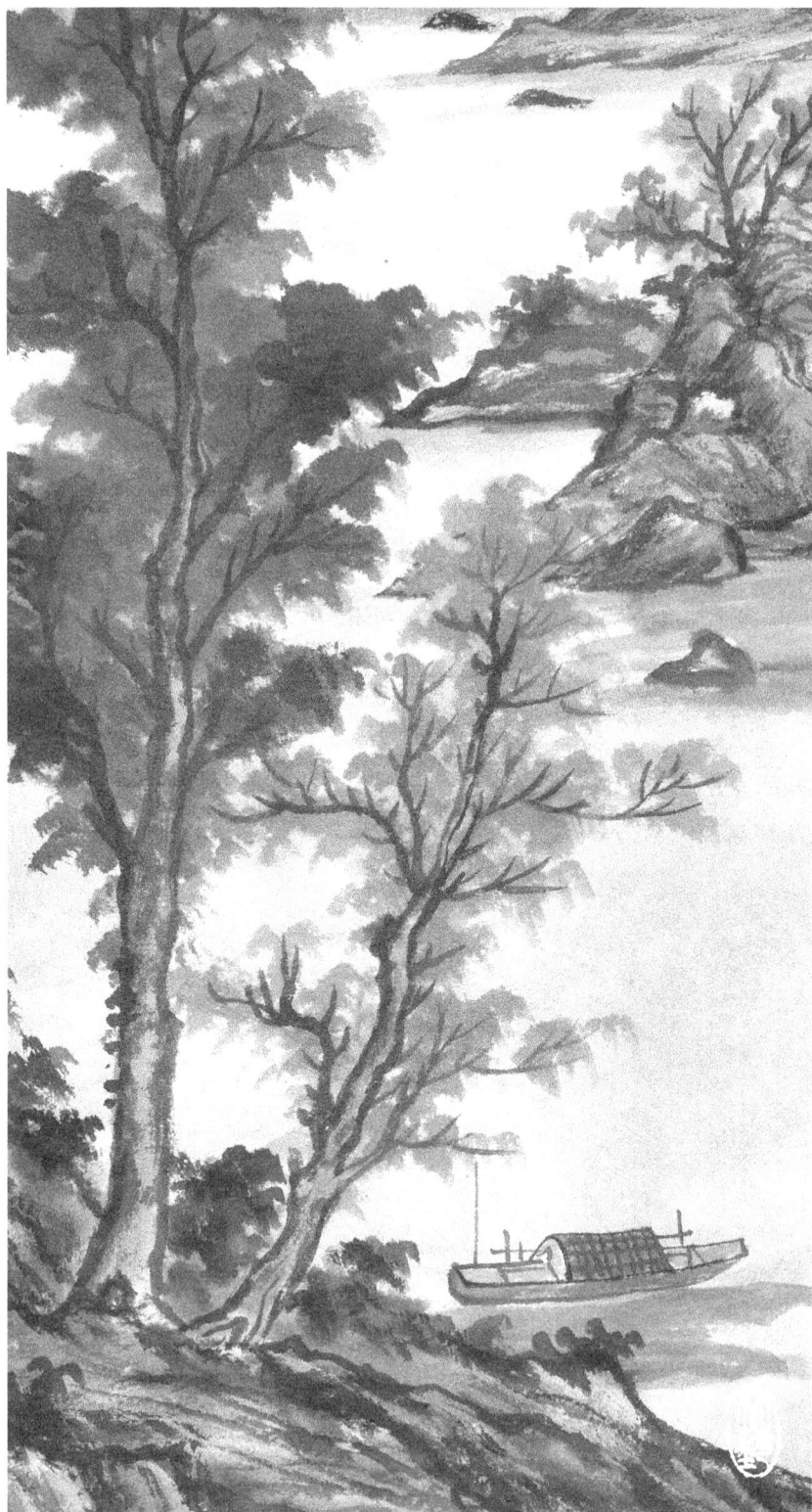

# CHAPTER TWENTY

On the thirteenth day, Liu and Pei Ke were traveling through a dense bamboo forest. Liu liked this road because it was a beautiful section of the journey and it gave Pei Ke a needed rest from climbing and descending the mountains. Liu knew Pei Ke's muscles needed exercising, but he also knew the body needed rest.

"Master, is it necessary for the patient to believe in acupuncture for it to work?"

"No, but you need to consider many factors when you are with a patient. First, you must build a doctor-patient relationship. Even if the patient outwardly indicates their disbelief in what you are doing, a patient's subconscious desire is to get well, otherwise, the patient would not come to see you. This desire to get well has its own energy, similar to the energy of someone who definitely believes. Never tell the patient that his belief that acupuncture does not work is wrong. When you do this, you are inserting a negative factor into his energy field, which the patient will sense. It is your job to acknowledge the patient's uncertainty and explain what you will do and relate the success you have had in using these techniques.

"Secondly, encourage the patient to give you feedback during the treatment process. The superior doctor makes decisions during the treatment process and if necessary, changes the prescription as the need arises. Remember, you are working with a system of energy and this system reacts differently for each person. Tap into the system to ensure it is doing what you anticipate it will do. Your treatment process is changing the energy of the patient and you need to make adjustments to your technique as the situation warrants.

"The third factor is your level of confidence in what you do. If you are not confident, the patient will sense it and this lack of confidence will have an effect on how soon the patient recovers. Your confidence level will increase through continual study and practice. Even to this day, I set aside time for studying and researching the various aspects of this art. I continually discover new ways to tap into the universal energy that keeps us all alive and healthy.

"The fourth factor is how you respond to a patient when he says he has been to other practitioners and still has the same problems. Though you acknowledge the person has been to another practitioner, never suggest that the previous practitioner was inferior. Doing so sets up doubt in the patient's mind about all practitioners.

"The fifth factor is the patient's own desire or lack of desire to solve his health problems. Sometimes a patient doesn't want to get well. Some individuals derive emotional benefit when they get attention from others. If the attention they receive is greater than the discomfort they experience, there may be little incentive for them to get well. Getting better requires them to give up the emotional benefit they receive from poor health. These individuals have a hidden agenda and an emotional blockage.

"The sixth factor concerns a fundamental human characteristic of wanting to believe there is hope in the treatment. We as doctors think we know everything about the human body and how it will respond. The feeling of hope has a certain type of energy. If you convey the feeling of hopelessness, the energy will change. You can actually see the change take place in someone's face. You can never be one hundred percent certain of the outcome of your treatments or the severity of any health care issue. There is always hope.

"The seventh factor is the immediacy of results. Many people try acupuncture to see if it works. Quite often, a patient does not understand the process needed to make changes in the energy system. You must get the patient well as quickly as possible, but progress is not always evident in the first visit. Progress depends on the individual's response to the treatment, the length of time he has had the problem, and the type of problem. The patient needs to be aware of this so that the treatment process can continue.

"The eighth factor in a patient's belief system is the information he obtains from others that you and your colleagues have treated. If the experience was favorable, the patient is more likely to have a favorable impression and expectations. As much as possible, leave the patient with a good impression of what you are trying to do.

"Sometimes the condition is so chronic that it will take many visits to fully balance the patient's internal energy. Be sure to mention this to the patient. It is important for the patient to understand that many years of accumulated pain may not go away instantly.

"The ninth factor is similar to having confidence in yourself, but deals with your own belief system. Do you believe you can heal others? Do you want to heal others? Many doctors are in this field for the wrong reasons. Greed and misguided goals have led them to covet the so-called good things in life at the expense of their patients. The energy of that feeling will eventually permeate to their patients. The patients will sense it and react negatively to the feeling."

"Master, being a doctor carries with it a tremendous amount of responsibility."

"Yes, Pei Ke, you should not take it lightly. Always put yourself in a position to understand your patient's point of view. He is the one who has put his trust in your hands. Do justice to that trust."

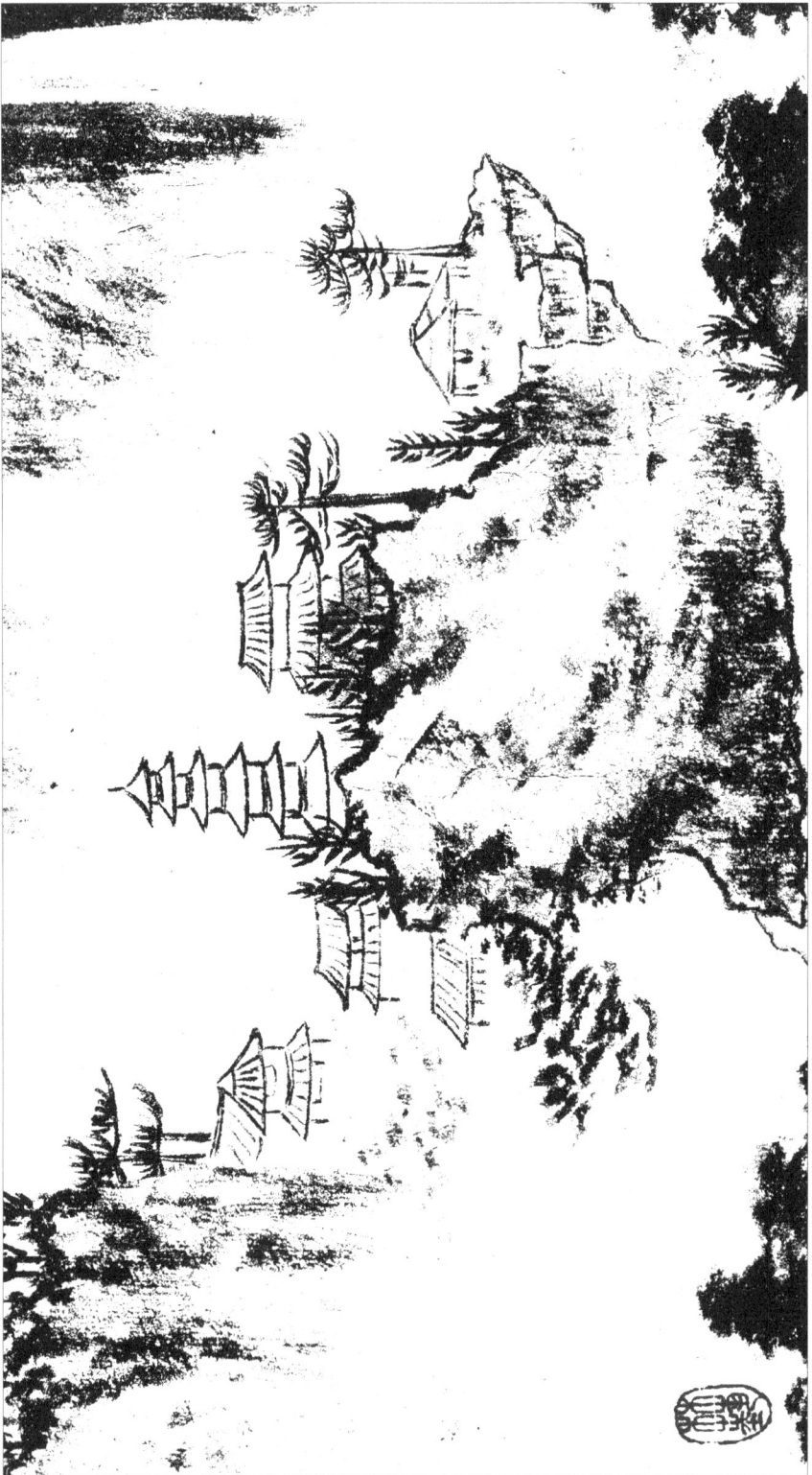

# CHAPTER TWENTY-ONE

Liu and Pei Ke continued their northerly journey toward Liu's ancestral birthplace. The farther they traveled, the harder it was for Liu to conceal his uneasiness from his student. He found Pei Ke watching him nervously on several occasions and so Liu tried hard to keep up the intensity of their lessons.

On the fourteenth day of travel, they arrived at the Monastery of the Living Lotus. From the monastery, one could see far into the distance. The view was spectacular, but the manner in which the buildings were situated made the place unique. Each building opened to a different direction, and each direction had a view of either a valley or a mountain or both.

There, the Buddhist monks practiced the original exercises brought from India by Boddirama. Liu had visited this monastery in the past. He was welcomed as if he was a member of the monastery. They also greeted Pei Ke with no hesitation. The monks found it surprising that Liu, at his age, had taken on another student.

"Pei Ke, you are free to explore. I want to discuss some things with the Abbot."

Many of the monks were cultivating the gardens. Each monk took responsibility for a certain area. Some cultivated the vegetables used in their traditional cooking, while others worked what appeared to be herbs. The monks everywhere bowed in greeting and Pei Ke bowed back to them. He strolled through the areas of the monastery, not looking for anything or anybody in particular, but absorbing everything he saw. This journey had been difficult so far, and dangerous, and he was beginning to value any moment of rest and serenity.

He found the main temple and asked permission from one of the monks to go inside. The temple was like most temples he had seen. The ornate richness of the decorations impressed Pei Ke. The walls were red, gold, and white. After spending a few minutes in the temple, Pei Ke returned to Liu. The master was sitting and talking with the Abbot. When the master saw him approach, he signaled for Pei Ke to join them.

"We will stay the night. The Abbot has graciously extended his welcome to us."

Pei Ke bowed to the monk, who in turn bowed to Pei Ke.

"I understand from Master Liu you are studying martial arts and medicine. Master Liu's family has a good reputation throughout this province. You are fortunate to study from him. He will teach you things in martial arts and medicine few people know. Study diligently. Maybe one day you will return and visit us again. You are always welcome here."

"Thank you. This is truly a beautiful place," Pei Ke said. "I feel so honored and fortunate to have this opportunity to be here. Everyone is happy and enjoying life, with little or no worries or stress. You must have many monks here at the monastery?"

"We have over a hundred monks living here. In addition, we take in about ten new initiates each year. Unfortunately, about half of each group departs within the year. The training is disciplined, but not torturous. Yet many lack the internal fortitude to stay with it. We try to identify the ones who we feel will have potential before they are accepted into the monastery, but we are not always successful.

"I have spoken with Master Liu about a husband and wife who live close to the monastery. Their financial generosity helped to establish this place. They continue to be benefactors these many years. They are elderly and both have some health concerns. Master Liu has agreed to see them. Ordinarily, I would not ask, nor would I divulge the situation, but the woman confided in me and asked if I thought anything could be done to help. She comes to the temple to pray quite often. I do not know medicine, but this may be a fortuitous situation for her. I sent one of the monks to their home to bring them here. Her situation is quite personal and embarrassing for her. When they come I will let the two of you have private time with them. While we are waiting for them to come, I can answer any questions you have."

"Are the monks free to leave the monastery at any time?"

"Yes and no." The Abbot made a face that Pei Ke was coming to recognize well. It indicated that he had asked a question that had a very complicated answer. Nothing was as simple as it seemed, apparently.

"As long as they want to be members of this sect," the Abbot said, "they are required to stay here at all times. There are some exceptions, such as family duties and other important matters. Of course, if there are specific things we need them to do away from the monastery, they will be allowed to go. In that case, we usually have more than one monk go together. If a monk decides to permanently leave these walls, we will spend some time discussing his decision with him. We have no hold on the monks. We cannot force them to stay. Once a monk has been here for a few years, it is highly unlikely he will want to leave. The training here, while very disciplined, is ideal for development of the eternal energy. Once a monk decides to leave, his decision is irrevocable; he will not be allowed to return. By then he would have experienced too much of the earthly ways of the outside. His wants and desires will have influence on the development of the other monks."

"I don't see any women in the monastery. Do you allow women here?"

"It would be a major distraction for us to have both men and women."

"Do more men or women come to the temple for devotion? I know my mother always went and my father seldom went, except when my mother forced him to go."

"The majority of our devout worshipers are women. They sometimes bring their husbands to keep them company. The men, however, are not as devout as the women. A woman's intuition and the feminine aspect bring them to Buddha. Of course, we believe all of us should pray to Buddha on a daily basis. Prayer and self sacrifice help purify our bodies."

The Abbot continued to answer questions until a young monk came to announce the arrival of the guests.

As the three of them walked toward the monastery, Liu and the Abbot were in deep conversation about some philosophical concepts, but Pei Ke paid little attention to what was being discussed. He was contemplating the feasibility of becoming a monk. The pros and cons went through his mind. Soon the cons won out over the pros. Being in such a beautiful place was intriguing, but its monotony was not for him. He had experienced too much of the outside world.

––––––––––––

The Abbot took them into a secluded room in the monastery and introduced Liu and Pei Ke to Gao Shi Fei and his wife Gao Mei Yi. After an exchange of introductions and pleasantries, the Abbot departed.

"As the Abbot had mentioned, my student Pei Ke is studying with me and has been with me on other cases. Please do not feel uncomfortable by his presence."

Liu walked over to the table where the couple was sitting and motioned for Pei Ke to sit with him.

"What can I do for you? The Abbot only told me you have some health concerns and that I might be of some help."

"It is more important for you to help my wife," said Mr. Gao. "She has suffered for many years."

"Mrs. Gao, how can I help?"

Tears rolled down her cheeks, as she looked first at Liu then at Pei Ke.

"I have had incontinence for many years and it is getting worse over time. I have to wear protective pads all the time. It is so embarrassing. I am afraid to go anywhere in case I have an accident. Is there anything you can do? I will take any help."

"I may be able to help. I first need to ask you a series of questions. Would you like for your husband to leave while I ask?"

"No. he knows everything already."

"Mrs. Gao, do you mind going over to the bed and lying down.

Liu helped her get up and walked with her to the bed. Holding her hand, he helped her lie down. He adjusted the pillow and put one of the extra pillows under her knees to take the pressure off her back.

"Master Liu, do you really think you can help me?"

"I think so, but you must answer my questions first. How long have you had this problem?"

"For about fifteen years now."

"How did it start?"

"I don't know."

"I have been practicing medicine most of my life. We need to work as a team. It is not me seeing you and it is not you seeing me. It is both of us brought together by divine intervention to solve a problem. The more information you can give me, the better I am able to diagnose the problem. You may find the trivial things seem unimportant to you, but, these small details allow me to differentiate one cause from another. Give me as much information as possible."

"I really don't know why it started. I suppose I first noticed it after my last child was born. It took me much longer to heal. I have had the problem ever since."

"How many children do you have?"

"We have six children, four girls and two boys. The last one was a boy and was born fifteen years ago."

"Did your mother have the same problem?"

"No, but she had other problems."

"Are your parents still alive?"

"No. My mother died from a stroke and my father was killed in a mountain climbing accident."

"Do you have any sisters who have the same problem?"

"I have two sisters and one brother and no one has this problem, at least not that I know of."

"What color is the urine when you urinate? Is it clear, pale or dark in color?"

"It is either clear or pale, depending on how much green tea I have had to drink."

"Do you have to urinate often?"

"Yes, quite often. At night, I need to get up at least two to three times. If I don't, I will have an accident. It feels like an urgency. It also feels as if my bladder is getting smaller and smaller each year. Is that possible?"

"I don't know if it is getting smaller, but something is causing this problem. Is there a difference in the amount of times you have to urinate between daytime and nighttime?"

"No, it's about the same. Of course, during the night I do not drink as much fluids as I would during the day. I am to the point that I don't want to drink much tea."

"Is there a burning sensation when you urinate?"

"No."

"Is there any particular smell to your urine?"

"No."

"Is there any blood in your urine?"

"No, I have never seen any blood."

"Do you always seem to urinate at the same time of the day or night?"

"No, there is no consistent time. I just have to urinate frequently."

"Do you feel bloated or swollen in your abdomen, ankles, or hands?"

"No."

"How old are you?"

"I'm fifty."

"Do you still have a monthly period?"

"No, it stopped two years ago."

"When you were having a period, was there a difference in your incontinence?"

"No, it was the same, just getting worse as I get older. Is my age the reason for this problem?"

"It could be, but I suspect a different reason. Do you have any abdominal pain?"

"No."

"Do you have recurring headaches, backache, vision problems, or pain in the knees?"

"I have occasional lower back pain and some shoulder pain, but it usually comes from lifting too much. Do you think the lifting has caused me to have the incontinence?"

"Probably not. How much sleep do you get at night?"

"I don't sleep as much as I used to, but I think I get enough that I am not tired during the day."

"Do you have any unusual taste in your mouth?"

"No."

"Do you consistently eat the same foods all the time?"

"No, but be sure to ask my husband that question."

"Do you have any problem with breathing, chills, fever, perspiration, or loss of appetite?"

"No, all those things are fine."

"Do you have a bowel movement at least once a day?"

"Yes."

"Mrs. Gao, I am going to feel your abdomen to see if there is anything unusual."

"Please do not press too hard. I don't want to urinate."

"Do you need to urinate now?"

"No, I went before I came."

"When you want to urinate, do you have any problem doing so?"

"No, I don't have any problem."

"Have you had any injuries to your abdomen?"

"No, why do you ask?"

"If there were scars across the abdomen or injuries to the abdomen, that could be a reason for the incontinence. Scars across the abdomen between the umbilicus and the pelvis tend to block the upward flow of Qi."

Liu pressed gently on the abdomen, feeling both sides and in the middle. When he pressed on the acupuncture point Qu Gu, Mrs. Gao had a slight jerking sensation. He pressed on the acupuncture point Shen Mai and Mrs. Gao quickly moved her foot in pain. He next touched the acupuncture point Bai Hui and got a similar reaction.

"Are those points uncomfortable?"

"Slightly, did you find something wrong?"

"No, you are fine."

He touched other acupuncture points on her legs, arms, and body but did not get a pain response.

"I am going to feel your pulses on both of your wrists. It will help me determine where the imbalances are in your body so that I can treat you."

Liu started on her right side and felt the pulses, making a mental note of what he found. Then he did the same on the left side.

"Mrs. Gao, please stick out your tongue."

Liu looked at the color of the tongue, color of the fur, markings on the tongue, and the thickness and width of the tongue. As he bent over to look at the tongue, he made note of the smell of her breath and body.

"Is it serious?" asked Mrs. Gao.

"Yes and no," Liu said. "Yes, for you it is a concern and it will get worse unless it is treated. The good news is that for most women, it is readily treatable with acupuncture and herbs. This problem is common to women who have had difficult labors or many children. It is a complicated diagnosis, since some of the signs and symptoms are conflicting.

"Because of the downward pressure taking place during childbirth, sometimes the bladder becomes weak and descends. In many cases, it is a Qi deficiency problem. As I said, I have also seen this when a woman has an injury to the abdomen or a deep scar that cuts across the centerline of the abdomen. You will see a change if you will allow me to do acupuncture and moxibustion. Would that be all right with you?"

"Of course, Master."

Liu took some needles from his sack, held them in a flame for a few minutes and then let them cool.

"This will not be painful. I need to put some needles into your abdomen."

Mrs. Gao arranged her clothes so Liu had a clear, unobstructed view of her abdomen. He covered up the unneeded areas so that she would feel comfortable. Then he inserted three needles in her abdomen and two needles on each leg.

"I am now going to put one needle in your scalp and then I will twist the needle. Tell me what you feel in your abdomen."

Liu gently inserted a needle into Mrs. Gao's scalp.

"I feel a slight sensation," said Mrs. Gao.

"Does it feel as if there is a pulling up sensation in your abdomen?"

"Yes, that's it. It feels as if something is being pulled up or stretched, or maybe lifted. It is strange, but it does not hurt."

"Pei Ke, I want you to watch how I am twirling this needle in Mrs. Gao's scalp. This is the method of tonification for this point. If I did a dispersion technique her incontinence may become worse."

Pei Ke watched intently as Liu twirled the needle.

"Pei Ke, bring my bag here. Mrs. Gao, I will do some moxibustion on the needles. Do you know what that is?"

"Yes, I have seen it done before. I understand it feels warm and very soothing."

"Yes. Most everyone likes it. In fact when I stop, patients usually ask me not to."

Liu reached into his bag and took out a long thin stick of moxa.

"Pei Ke, there is more than one way to use moxa. Quite often the moxa is put on the skin or on the end of the needle. When it has been lit, than the heat penetrates into the acupuncture point. I prefer to roll up the loose moxa in rice paper. If it is tightly rolled you can hold it like a stick. This allows you to adjust the quantity of heat. Now, take this moxa stick and hold it over the flame until it glows."

Pei Ke took the round stick and held it over the flame as Liu continued to examine Mrs. Gao.

"Pei Ke, is the moxa stick ready?"

"Yes, Master, it is glowing."

"Come over here and hold it over these acupuncture points. Move the moxa stick up and down over the needle site. She will feel the heat increasing and decreasing. This technique increases the amount of Qi along the Conception Vessel Meridian and tonifies the energy. It will substantially help her incontinence. Mrs. Gao will tell you if it is too hot."

Pei Ke took the moxa stick and held it over the points as indicated.

"Mr. Gao, while he is doing the treatment, we can talk for a few minutes."

"Is she going to be all right?" asked Mr. Gao.

"Yes, I think so. I will give her a prescription for some herbs, which she will need to take for a few days. I think this will help. You will also need to do the moxibustion on some points for her. I will tell you which ones later. Now, do you have any health issues that we can take care of tonight?"

"My main complaint is that I have hemorrhoids. They've been bothersome for many years and are quite uncomfortable. I also have ringing in both ears."

"Mr. Gao, please sit in the chair."

Liu went through the same diagnostic procedure with Mr. Gao as he did with Mrs. Gao, always making mental notes of the signs and symptoms. He felt the pulses.

"Your wife mentioned you have a particular interest in some foods."

"Yes, I love to eat hot and spicy foods, but there seems to be a correlation between the food I eat and my hemorrhoids. Is that true?"

"In Chinese medicine, there are correlations between the food we eat and the way we feel. There are also correlations between many different aspects of our life and our health. With you there does seem to be a correlation. Let me look at your tongue and feel your pulses."

Liu felt the pulses again and then looked at Mr. Gao's tongue.

"Master, can you tell me what is wrong?"

"It appears that your condition is not serious, but it is quite uncomfortable for you. We can treat this problem, but you must substantially reduce the amount of spicy food you eat if you want this problem to go away completely."

"In other words you are telling me that I can have my spicy foods and suffer the hemorrhoids, or do away with the spicy foods and possibly have the hemorrhoids go away."

"Yes."

"I can never have spicy foods again?"

"I didn't say it that way; you can have a little every once in a while. You will have to see what your body can tolerate."

"Why did my body get to this condition?"

"It is probably due to an excess diet of spicy foods. Think of it this way. Suppose we slowly pour water into a cup. As we pour more and more water into the cup, the water level will rise to the brim until even one more drop causes the water to overflow. That is a threshold level. Once your body has gone past the threshold level, it can no longer support that level of water. You have gone past your threshold level for spicy foods.

"This overabundance also happens with people who have allergies. They can tolerate a certain plant or food until they reach the threshold level for their bodies for that particular item. I have seen this in people who were raised in a certain part of the country and then moved to another part of the country. The first year or two they are fine, but over time they have worse and worse sinus problems as the cup of what they can tolerate as an allergen fills up to the threshold level. The important thing to remember is that allergies are easily treated and people do not need to suffer."

"You mean you can successfully treat allergies?"

"Yes, I have treated numerous people with seasonal and food allergies. Many of these people were truly miserable."

"I have a friend who suffers each spring and autumn with seasonal allergies. How many acupuncture sessions would it take to solve his problem?"

"Sometimes the allergy is straightforward and very easy to solve. Other times, it is quite complex and would take a number of visits. The underlying cause of the allergies, quite often, is lung energy or a liver energy problem. Of course, it does not mean there is anything wrong with the patient's lungs or liver. It only means that there is an imbalance along the meridian system associated with the lung and liver."

"Master, we are simple people. We do not understand all you have said. You put needles in my wife to help her. Are there acupuncture points you can use to help me with my hemorrhoids?"

"Of course, and I will do so in a moment. First, I must see to your wife. Mrs. Gao, how do you feel?"

"I am feeling better, thank you. I have a nice warm feeling."

Liu took the needles out and helped Mrs. Gao to a chair.

"Do you feel all right?"

"Yes. Yes, of course."

"Mr. Gao, please lie down. You mentioned ringing in your ears."

"Yes, I have had this problem for a couple of years."

"Is the ringing in one ear or is it in both ears?"

"It is in both ears."

"Is it constant ringing or does it come and go?"

"It comes and goes, but I have not been able to identify why it starts and stops."

"Does the ringing in the ears happen at any particular time of the day or night?"

"No, it is quite random and it lasts for varying periods of time."

"What other problems do you have when you hear the ringing?"

"None, Master."

"Do you have a backache?"

"Yes, quite often. It comes and goes. There is a feeling across my back, almost like a tightness."

"Do you have headaches when you have the ringing in the ears?"

"No, I seldom have headaches."

"Do you ever have a strange, different, or unique taste in your mouth?"

"No."

"Do you get dizzy with the ringing in the ears?"

"Yes. Often when the ringing is severe, I will get dizzy. Sometimes I have to sit down or lay down because I feel I will fall or collapse."

Liu once again felt the pulses and looked at Mr. Gao's tongue.

"Mr. Gao, ringing in the ears can be either an excess or a deficiency condition. From what you indicated and what I have felt on the pulses, you have a deficiency condition. The good news is this problem, like the hemorrhoid problem, it is solvable. The bad news is you will need more than one treatment."

"How many treatments will I need?"

"It is hard to tell now until you have had one or two treatments. Herbal formulations may also help with this problem."

After Mr. Gao lay down, Liu inserted needles into various acupuncture points. One of the needles went into the same acupuncture point used for Mrs. Gao. One needle went into his abdomen and Liu twisted the needle to tonify the energy. The others went into the arms and legs.

"Master, I see you are using some of the same points for both patients," Pei Ke said.

"Yes, a couple of the points are the same, but for different reasons. Both patients have an imbalance that I am trying to correct. If I can do that, they both will have favorable results. You will learn from experience that acupuncture points can be used for a multitude of different problems depending on how the energy is unbalanced. Remember it is best for the patient to first have a diagnosis. Then choose the points carefully. Do not always choose the same points for the same problem. Yes, some people will get better but your outcome will be far superior if you rely on the diagnosis. That is one of the problems with some practitioners. They expect the same points to always be able to treat the same problem. A good example would be headaches. If ten people had a headache in the same area of their head there could easily be ten different acupuncture prescriptions and ten different herbal prescriptions. Basing the treatment protocol on the underlying cause is far superior to basing the treatment protocol on the symptom. The headache is the symptom, not the cause."

"Will both these patients have to take herbs?"

"Yes, but as I just indicated, the herb formulas will be different because the differential diagnosis is unique for each of them. It wouldn't make sense to give them the same herbs unless they had the same diagnosis. Now, let me finish."

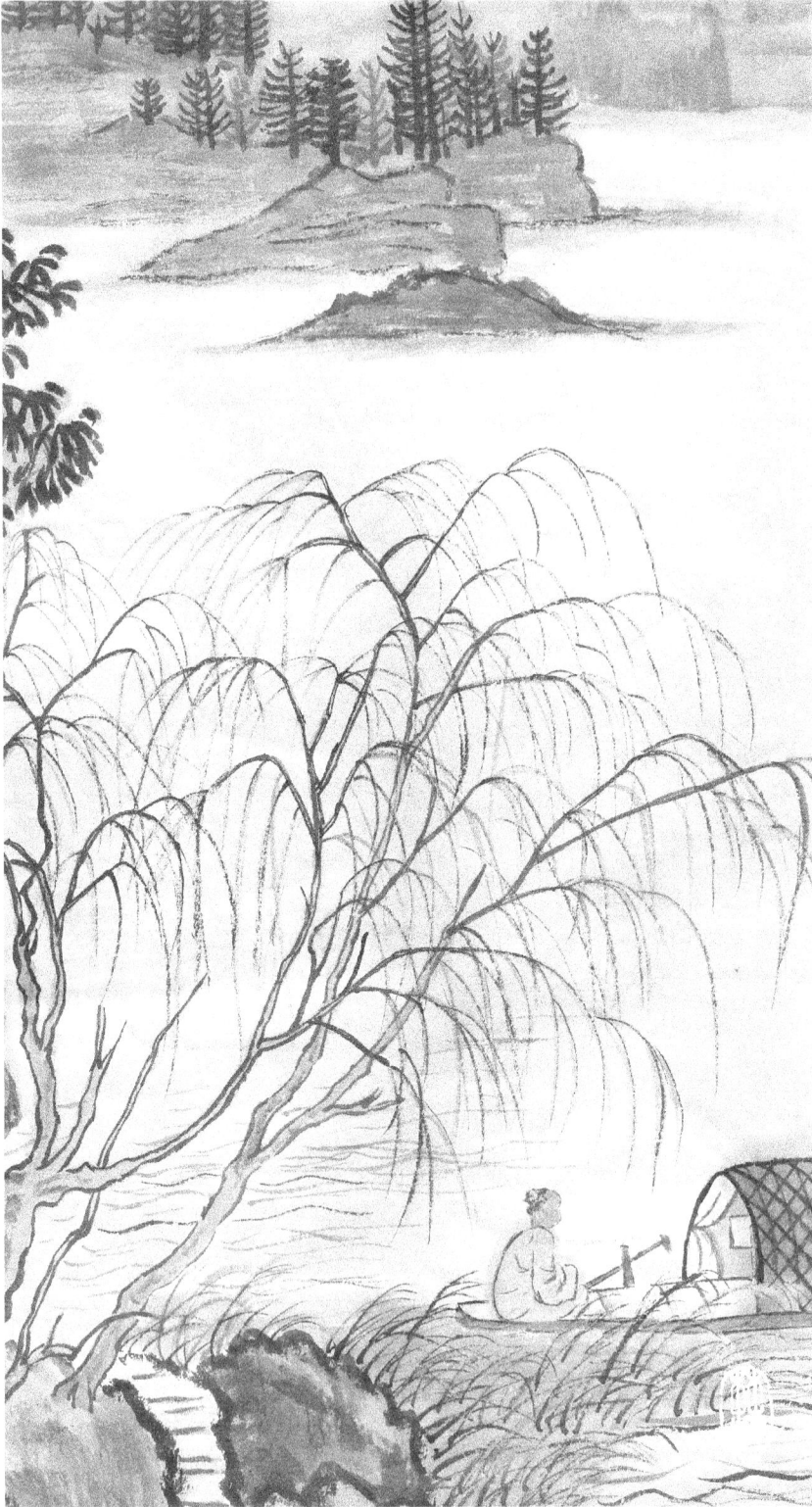

# CHAPTER TWENTY-TWO

On the fifteenth day, they stayed with Huo De Sheng, a well-known painter and calligrapher. Not only was he renown in the arts, but he was also a representative of the Imperial Government. His dealings with the people in his district were always correct and proper, though he was known for carrying formality to the extreme. Despite this, everyone trusted Huo.

"You will like Huo De Sheng," Liu said as they approached. "He studied painting, calligraphy, and poetry some time ago. Since learning from me, he has gone on to study from others, but we have kept in touch over the years. His wife is an excellent cook and makes a superb tofu and garlic dish, which she always serves when they have visitors. Maybe she will serve it tonight."

"How soon before we get there?"

"We will be there before the sun sets."

Pei Ke tried to put thoughts of food from his head and asked, "Did Huo study martial arts or did he only study the literary arts?"

"Huo studied martial arts for a short time. His son is studying martial arts from Wang."

"You mean Mr. Wang who owns the teahouse?"

"Yes, Wang excels in external martial arts. Huo's son helps in the kitchen in exchange for learning Wang's system of martial arts. Huo studied martial arts for a short time with me, but his main focus was learning how to paint bamboo. There are many techniques for painting bamboo, but he wanted to learn mine. He has done some beautiful paintings over the years. His fame has spread and many people have purchased his scrolls. He has donated some of his work to the surrounding temples. When you look at his bamboo paintings, you will see both a depth to the painting and a unique liveliness. One day he will be famous for his artwork. I know you will enjoy visiting with Huo and his wife."

"It must be nice to afford art work," Pei Ke said without thinking.

"You would like to have some artwork?"

"Of course," Pei Ke said.

"Then I will teach you how to paint, and you can have all the artwork you want," Liu said.

They continued throughout the day, stopping only to rest and get water. He was once again amazed at the difference only a few short miles made in the way the land looked.

"Master, what is it like in other areas? I know you have been many places and have studied from many teachers."

"Each area is different and, of course, each area has its customs and dialect. I have been as far south as Wu Tang Mountain. Legend tells us that is the birthplace of Tai Chi Chuan. The mountain is unique. There is a tremendous amount of energy in that place. I have felt similar feelings in other places, but it is particularly strong for me at that location.

"The area around the mountain is home to many who come to meditate and cultivate their internal energy. I spent some time traveling around the mountain and met quite a few of its inhabitants. Some excellent martial artists live there. I watched some of them practice. It is a joy to see the beauty and fluidity of their arts, some of which exist only in this area. Many of these masters teach only one or two students in their lifetime."

"Is it possible for us to go there?"

"We could travel there some time in the future. My main concern now is reaching my home."

"Yes, of course, Master. I didn't mean for us to go now. It would be nice to see other things and other places."

"I have been as far west as Chengdu in Sichuan Province. The Monastery of the Precious Light, which is located in Chengdu, is probably one of the most beautiful monasteries I have ever seen. Sichuan Province is famous for its hot and spicy foods. I have had some dishes that were so spicy they were almost impossible to eat. The local people laughed that I could not tolerate the spiciness. There is a particularly good place to eat, similar to Wang's teahouse, just inside the city area. As you sip tea, you can hear musicians playing the local Sichuan opera music. It is both relaxing and enjoyable.

"Sichuan is also the natural habitat of the panda bear. I think you would find these animals quite interesting. I actually saw one of them while I was there. They are much smaller than regular bears and are not very aggressive. They reside mainly in the mountains and are sometimes difficult to locate. Their diet is almost exclusively bamboo leaves."

"And beyond Chengdu, Master?"

"About sixty miles West of Chengdu, the countryside becomes very mountainous and travel is quite limited. Some of the mountains, like Gongga Mountain, which is southwest of Chengdu, are over seven thousand feet high. The areas to the north, west, and southwest of Chengdu are sparsely populated. I do not know what lies beyond that. My main intent was to spend some time at the monastery in Chengdu, meditating and talking with the monks. Their hospitality was truly genuine.

"About a hundred miles south of Chengdu is Leshan. There a two-hundred-thirty-foot sculpture of Buddha has been carved out of rock, and a little bit farther is Emei Mountain, which has many monasteries. You would like that area, as it is peaceful and relaxing, good for meditating.

"Travels eastward have taken me to Shanghai, which is on the coast of the great ocean. It was there I saw my first foreigner."

"Master, I have never seen a foreigner. I understand their eyes are round and they talk with a strange accent, dress in strange clothes, have very absurd customs and mannerisms, and smell funny. Is that true?"

"From our point of view, their manner of speaking and dress do seem ridiculous, but I am sure they feel the same way about us. Some people in Shanghai have no tolerance for these outsiders and want nothing more than for them to go. I personally feel everything has its place. As long as they do us no harm, they are free to come and go.

"I can imagine what it would be like if I were in their country. The customs and mannerisms would be entirely different. Everyone would be looking at me and wondering all sorts of things. I would be uncomfortable. As long as the emperor sees fit to have them here and they don't affect me, I am tolerant."

"What is Shanghai like?"

"It is a very large city, possibly one of the largest cities in China.

"The emperor has become influenced by the West and is allowing the Westerners to come to this country for a reason. Many of them stay in a section of Shanghai reserved for foreigners. We as a country have thought of ourselves as being the center of the world for five thousand years. It comes as a shock to know other places have advanced just as we have, but in another direction. Maybe someday we will go to Shanghai."

"I would enjoy that, Master." Pei Ke looked around, wondering if he would see things differently if he were as well traveled as his master.

"How far north have you traveled?" he asked.

"I have been as far north as Beijing. Some of my former students live there. Many good martial art teachers live in Beijing and you can learn everything that you could ever want to learn. In fact, you could spend a lifetime just in Beijing, learning.

"The Forbidden City, where the emperor resides, is in Beijing. His many servants help him with his personal affairs and help him manage the affairs of state. He spends most of his time behind the walls of the huge palace compound, as though he is a captive within his own country. It is forbidden for common folk to enter the Forbidden City, so I do not know what is inside those walls, but it is no concern of mine. His decrees have little or no effect on me."

"Master, I understand a great wall stretches from east to west to keep out invaders from the north. Have you seen it?"

"Yes. It is like a dragon stretching across China from east of Beijing all the way to Jiayuguan in West Central China. The wall was constructed to take advantage of the terrain of the countryside. It is wide enough to allow both troops and horses on the top.

"From any one guard tower you can see the towers both to the left and right. In this way, communication flows along the wall from one tower to the next. It is built of materials that are common to the area. Where it is mountainous, they used mostly rock. Where rock was not that common, earth was used as much as possible. In some places, the wall is over forty feet high and more than thirty feet wide at the base. Thousands of workers were conscripted to build the wall in sections. During the reign of Huang Di, he ordered the wall be joined together to what it is today. Sections of the wall are missing now, but the foundation is still present. You can imagine how many workers died before the wall was completed. I have only seen a small part of the wall, close to Beijing."

"Master, if you didn't live at the temple where would you like to live?"

"I probably would not live in a big city. The peacefulness of the rural areas is too enticing. The people are more genuine, and the way of life is in keeping with the philosophy of the Tao. Still, it is nice to visit the large cities and see what they have to offer. There are many things to do, but most of the things that the people get involved in are external to true happiness. The city only satisfies the immediate external desire—never the true internal path of enlightenment.

"In Beijing and Shanghai, I have many friends and I have fond memories of long philosophical discussions on painting, martial arts, medicine, and poetry. It would be nice to visit with them once again."

Just before sunset, Liu and Pei Ke turned off the road and walked the short distance to Huo's house. Pei Ke was really looking forward to meeting Huo and his wife. Dogs announced their arrival and the front door opened just as they approached the house.

"It's Master Liu," shouted the woman who stood in the doorway. She came out the door to bow and greet Liu. Seconds later, Huo De Sheng emerged and greeted Liu with great respect.

"Master, you are traveling with a companion," Huo said.

"Yes, this is Pei Ke. He is a student of mine and is accompanying me on this trip home."

Pei Ke bowed first to Huo, then to his wife.

"Come in," said Huo. "Have you eaten?"

"No, not yet."

As they stepped inside, Liu could sense someone watching him, but he could not tell if it was time for something to happen. In the past, he often could tell the true intent of people just by feeling the energy they emitted, much like the energy one feels when walking into a crowded room. For now, the energy was neutral.

"My wife is preparing her famous tofu and garlic dish," Huo said. "You are just in time."

"Thank you," Liu said. "May we also stay with you this evening?"

"Of course you may. It would be an honor. I have told you many times that our home is always available to you. Come, let us sit for a while."

"If you will excuse me," said Mrs. Huo. "I must attend to the meal and prepare your room."

"Mrs. Huo," Liu said, looking at his apprentice firmly. Pei Ke had been in the process of sitting and now froze. "Pei Ke is learning to cook. Would it be possible for him to watch you prepare the food? Maybe you can share some of your culinary experience with him."

"Of course," Mrs. Huo said.

Before Pei Ke could utter a word, Mrs. Huo turned to him.

"It is good that men learn to cook. Come with me and leave the two of them to talk."

Reluctantly Pei Ke turned and followed her down the hallway. As they walked to the kitchen area, Pei Ke noticed the many paintings on the walls, including a bamboo scene done by Liu. Alongside Liu's scroll was one done by Huo. Pei Ke stopped for a moment to compare the two paintings. Even though Huo had mastered the technique, it was easy to tell the master from the student.

"Mrs. Huo," Pei Ke said when they arrived at the kitchen. "Master Liu told me of your famous tofu and garlic dish." He looked around the large, well-equipped kitchen.

"Yes, I only make it when we have guests. My husband would like it more often but it is a special event when someone comes to visit. I started preparing it this morning because it takes a while to prepare. The tofu is ordinary, but the ingredients in the sauce are what make this dish special.

"First, you take soy sauce and add sesame seed oil. Then add garlic, rice wine vinegar, some special spices, followed by a little hot pepper sauce. Mix the ingredients. After the sauce has set for a while, pour it over the tofu and generously sprinkle chopped, fresh spring onions on as well. It can be eaten either hot or cold, but Master Liu prefers it hot, so I will heat it and sprinkle the spring onions on just before serving it."

Pei Ke looked at the spices but did not recognize any of them.

"The tofu without this special sauce would be tasty. With the special spices, a great dish now becomes an outstanding meal, and a great compliment to the other dishes."

"Mrs. Huo, I have a question?"

"Of course."

"You only prepare this tofu dish when you have guests. Is that correct?"

"Yes. I start early in the day so that the sauce can set awhile before it is used."

"Are you having any guests besides Master Liu and me for dinner tonight?"

"No, I don't foresee anyone else coming to visit today."

Pei Ke looked at Mrs. Huo who looked back and smiled.

"Mrs. Huo, if you only make this dish when you have guests, and it takes some time for the sauce, you must have known we were coming before we actually arrived."

"My husband and I are Taoist. We meditate for a couple hours every morning. We both tap into the universal energy and knowledge when we meditate. Our individual energy becomes one energy for us. In essence, we are one with the universal energy of the Tao-part of the universal energy that is made up of thoughts and actions. If we meditate on a particular subject, topic, or upcoming event we can understand what lies ahead for us. This energy guides us in our daily activities and is responsible for everything we do during the day. Has Master Liu taught you Qi Gong?"

"Yes, he has taught me the fourteen basic Qi Gong exercises. We practice it almost every day."

Pei Ke could see a smile on Mrs. Huo's face, but he could not detect what the smile indicated. Was she smiling because she knew something that he did not know or was she smiling because she knew he was intrigued by her knowledge? Maybe she was smiling because she knew it would take an inordinate amount of time and practice for him to get to her level of understanding.

So, he thought to himself. Mrs. Huo knew that we were coming before we actually arrived. That could be why Master knows what other martial artists will do before they actually do it. What a gift to have and to cherish.

—————

When it was time for dinner, the four of them sat at a round table. Mrs. Huo served hot dishes and cold dishes, spicy dishes and bland dishes. The tofu and garlic dish was truly the highlight of the meal. After the dinner, while the servants took care of the kitchen, they had hot green tea.

"Huo, last time I saw you, your shoulder was bothering you. Is it better?'

"Yes, Master, you fixed my shoulder, but as age advances we seem to have more and more aches and pains. If you could do some of your magic on us, we would appreciate it."

"Of course. Do you mind if Pei Ke assists me? He is in training and I would like him to watch. He will hold everything you say in strict confidence."

"Master," Mrs. Huo said, "Let me talk with the servants and make sure your room is ready for the evening. We can visit later. Thank you for taking care of my husband. Again, we are indebted to you. Every time you come, we ask you to work."

"It is not work for me. I derive much pleasure and satisfaction from helping humanity. I believe that should be the primary reasons to enter into the healing art."

"But Master, you never charge any money, nor do you accept gifts."

"I have few needs other than a little food and a place to sleep for the night. My meditation and martial arts keep me balanced with the universal Tao."

As Pei Ke listened, he thought how poor his family had been. They were never able to afford anything other than a little food and a place to sleep. Of course, others had less food and less of a place to live. He was fortunate to have what he had. No matter how bad his circumstances might be, others had it worse. He caught himself feeling proud that he had had such a sage thought, one his master might have said.

"Master, let's go to the sleeping quarters where we can have some privacy," Huo said.

Pei Ke noticed how elegant the house was. He had only seen the outer waiting room, kitchen, and eating area, but the rest of the house was filled with fine furnishings and beautiful art. As they entered the sleeping quarters, Huo went over to the bed and sat down.

"What seems to be your problem?" Liu asked.

"A couple of months ago I hurt my back while chopping wood. Usually the servants chop the wood, but they were busy and I foolhardily decided to do it myself. I felt pain in my lower back later that day. It was not too bad then, it was more a feeling of stiffness. The next day, the pain was much worse and I could feel the pain going down the outside of my right leg to my calf muscles. It is difficult to sleep at night, since I cannot get in a comfortable position. The pain is constant, but varies in intensity during the day. When I stand from a seated position, the pain grabs me in the back and leg. If I turn a certain direction the pain is more intense."

"Pei Ke, do you remember what the process is when we treat patients?"

"Yes, Master."

"What is the first part of that process?"

"The first part is to inspect the patient, which includes observation of his spirit and vitality; observation of the color or lack of color in the patient; observation of his overall appearance; observation of the various sense organs; and observation of the patient's tongue."

"Which one is the most important?"

"Master, they are all important, for they give clues to the patient's underlying problem."

"Do you observe anything unusual with Mr. Huo?"

Pei Ke looked for a few minutes and asked Huo to stick out his tongue. He carefully looked at Huo's tongue.

"Master, Mr. Huo's tongue is a little dark, maybe purple in color. Other than that, I don't see anything unusual with him.

Liu turned to Huo. "Do you mind standing and walking across the room for us?"

Huo stood up and Pei Ke noticed instantly his difficulty in doing so. When Huo walked, he clearly favored one leg over the other.

"Master, he is leaning to one side."

"Yes. Now, what are the second and third processes?"

"The second process is listening and smelling. The third process is inquiring about the symptoms."

"When we inquire, what should we ask?"

"We need to ask about chills, perspiration, appetite, defecation and urination, pain, and sleep habits. If it is a woman, we need to ask about her menstrual cycle."

Liu nodded and turned to Huo with a gleam in his eyes. "As I am sure you've guessed, I need to ask you some questions. Try to answer them as accurately as possible. Do you have any problem with excessive perspiration or changes in your appetite?"

"No, Master."

"Has the pain in your back and leg ever gone away completely?"

"Yes, twice, the pain has left for a couple of days, but then it returned."

"What made the pain come back?"

"I lifted something heavy and felt the pain in my back."

"Is the pain more intense at a particular time of the day or night?"

"I have not really thought about it that way. It is probably worse when I lie down at night or when I am resting. Usually it is the way I stand or sit that makes the difference."

"The pain and discomfort is on the right side. Has there ever been any pain or discomfort on the left side?"

"No, the pain is always on the right side. The left side only feels a little stiff. I think I favor it over the other and it compensates for the right and throws my balance off, which makes the left side of my back stiff."

"Is the pain worse when you walk or when you are standing or sitting?"

"The pain is constant. It grabs when I turn or move in certain directions. It really hurts when I stand from a sitting position. It eases up after I have been standing and walking for awhile."

"Is there anything else I should know?"

"No. It just hurts."

"Do you have any kidney pain? There is a strong correlation between an imbalance in kidney energy and low back pain."

"No, I have no kidney pain."

"In Chinese medicine, excessive sexual activities deplete kidney energy and make the back weak, resulting in lower back pain."

"I remember you telling me that once before, but that is not a problem, especially since I hurt my back."

"Do you have any pain or problem with urination?"

"No."

"What color is your urine?"

"Clear with a slight yellow color. It has been normal all my life."

"Do you have any problem with bowel movements?"

"No, they are normal. I am occasionally a little constipated, but I see nothing that would be associated with my back pain."

"Is there any pain or discomfort on the bottom of your feet or on the top of your head?"

"No, everything is normal." He smiled suddenly. "Of course, my wife thinks I am hard-headed. Is there a cure for that?"

"Have you been fearful in the recent past?" Liu asked, smiling as well.

"No, everything is fine. I have no enemies that I know of and we live in harmony with the Tao. We take care of our servants. We have close friends with whom we associate on a continuous basis. There is no reason for me to be fearful of anything."

"Do you crave any particular foods?"

"No, but I prefer my wife's cooking over the cooking we get at the night markets."

"Do you have any particular lingering taste in your mouth?"

"No, other than the normal bad taste one has in the morning."

"Pei Ke, what is the fourth process we need to do with Mr. Huo?"

"The fourth process is palpation of the pulses and palpation of the body for sore points."

Liu felt Huo's pulses.

"Pei Ke, I want you to feel his pulses. He has a wiry pulse, which is an indication of a pain problem. It is usually associated with the Liver and Gallbladder Meridians."

Pei Ke felt the pulses as Liu had instructed and after a few minutes, he could discern the difference in the various pulses, including the wiry pulse on the Liver Meridian.

Liu continued the palpation process by applying pressure in the inguinal area, buttocks, and medial aspect of the leg just below the knee. Huo indicated that each area was sore. Liu then applied pressure on the Tai Chong, Yang Ling Quan, and Huan Tiao acupuncture points. Huo indicated they were all sore. Liu palpated other areas of Huo's abdomen and body. None of the other areas he palpated were sore.

Finally, Liu said, "Based on what we have found and what you have told us, stagnation of Blood and Qi is causing this problem. The stagnation is due to over exertion or a pulled muscle in your lower back. I will treat you to specifically relieve the pain and help eliminate the stagnation."

Liu had Huo lay on his side and then inserted needles into He Gu, Tai Chong, Yang Ling Quan, Huan Tiao, the urinary, bladder, and conception vessel points on the lower back, and numerous Ah Shi points on the leg and buttocks. Pei Ke watched intently, trying to understand the logic behind the choice of points. He knew energy collected at points and when it did, the point quite often would be sore. He surmised that Liu was using both the sore points on the meridian system and the Ah Shi points to correct the problem. He would remember this for future reference. He saw Huo relax as the muscle tightness in his legs and back started to ease. A few minutes later, Liu asked Huo some questions about his pain and then inserted some more needles. Thirty minutes later, he took out the needles and had Huo stand up.

"How do you feel now?"

"There is still some pain when I stand, but it is much better than it was before. Are there any herbs I can take to help?"

"Yes, there are herbs which will help promote the circulation of Qi and Blood and relieve the pain. I will write the prescription before leaving and you can take it to the herbalist. You may need more than one treatment to resolve this problem. Be sure to finish all of the herbs."

"Master, I want to thank you very much. We are always indebted to you, but I wonder if it would it be too much of a problem if you could help my wife? She is going through the change of life. One minute she is hot and another minute she is cold, and she perspires quite profusely."

"Of course, I will see her. Pei Ke, do you have any questions about this treatment process with Mr. Huo?"

"No, Master. I understood what you are doing and some of the logic, but I find it difficult to remember all the information. I presume it just takes years of clinical experience and practice."

"Yes, studying is important, but there is no substitute for clinical experience. Each time you have a different patient, you will remember what you did to help that patient. You may not remember each patient or the exact protocol you used, but the accumulation of experience will help you to be an outstanding practitioner."

"Master, how many years have you been doing medicine?"

"Most of my adult life. I have been fortunate to have more than one teacher, all of whom were willing to share their clinical experience and knowledge. Without these teachers, I would not know what I know today."

"Master, let me find my wife," said Huo. "She wants to talk to you about her problems." He sighed contentedly. "It is amazing how relaxing this session has been and how much better I am feeling. Thank you again, Teacher."

Huo walked away and Liu turned to Pei Ke.

"You had a nice talk with Mrs. Huo. Do you find her fascinating?"

"Master, she is more than fascinating. She seems to have transcended some earthly ties and is truly part of the universal Tao. Did she study from you?"

"Yes, she and her husband studied Qi Gong and meditation from me. Some people have a gift from the universe. They are lucky when they discover that gift and cultivate it. The human mind and body is capable of doing and accomplishing feats that seem both impossible and unreal. We have an unlimited capacity to develop our potential. All we need is guidance. You have the capacity to be truly great in something. Decide what it is you want to master and strive for it. Once mastered, it will comfort you for the rest of your life."

"Do you have any insight into what I should do, Master?"

"Pei Ke, that is entirely up to you. Look within yourself and try to discover what is most important to you."

As Liu was talking, Mrs. Huo entered the room.

"Master, my husband feels so much better. He has been complaining for quite some time. Thank you for helping him."

"I understand you have some health issues too. Maybe we can be of help. Is it all right if Pei Ke assists me?"

"Of course. The change of life has come upon me and I am experiencing some uncomfortable symptoms." She looked at the two men. "Who will be doing the acupuncture?"

"I will," Liu said. "He will be watching my technique. Please explain the symptoms."

"I have hot flashes during the day and evening. The evening ones are worse. My monthly periods ended two years ago and the hot flashes are getting worse. When they come, I perspire profusely. At night, my nightgown and pillow are soaked. Sometimes I am so hot I throw off the covers. A few minutes later I am cold and have to pull the covers back on me. This whole process of change is depriving me of a good night's sleep. I am putting on weight, which has never been an issue for me in the past. Also, my appetite is not as good as it used to be."

"I need to ask you some questions."

"I was sure you would," she said, smiling at Pei Ke.

Liu went through the four diagnostic methods of inspection, listening and smelling, inquiring as to the nature of the problem, and palpation. Pei Ke noted how consistent this process was from one patient to another, never omitting one of the steps.

After palpating Mrs. Huo's abdomen and feeling her pulses, Liu turned to Pei Ke.

"Pei Ke, this is a common problem for many women. Unless treated with acupuncture and Chinese herbs, it could continue for a couple of years. Fortunately, there are a number of acupuncture points we can choose, and a combination of these points will help relieve the symptoms. As I have told you before, combining the acupuncture with the herbs will be the most effective."

Liu put the needles in a flame for a few seconds and then let them cool for a few minutes.

"The first acupuncture point for this problem is San Yin Jiao. This point is the crossing point for the Spleen, Kidney, and Liver Meridians. These are important meridians for dealing with women's health care issues. The second point is Tai Xi, which treats both male and female problems. In this case, the points help regulate and balance her energy. The third and fourth points are Gong Sun and Nei Guan. These two points when used together have a calming effect on the chest and upper body. Many times when women are going through the change of life, they are tense or have anxiety. I will also use Zu San Li because it is on the Stomach Meridian, and the Spleen Meridian and Stomach Meridian are related."

Pei Ke listened as Liu went on to describe the other acupuncture points he was going to use and why he was choosing those specific points. After the explanation, Pei Ke watched as Liu inserted needles into the points.

"Mrs. Huo, I have put all the needles in. How do you feel?

"I feel calmer now. Thank you."

"Before I leave, I will write a prescription for you. Please take it to the herbalist. Be sure and take the herbs faithfully."

"Yes, Master. I will follow your directions."

"If possible, ask the herbalist if he knows an acupuncturist. You would benefit from more acupuncture treatments."

"How many do you think I will need?"

"That will depend on how well you respond to them and how well the herbs work. It is difficult for me to say unless I have done more treatments and could see how you progressed with your symptoms. But you should start feeling better now."

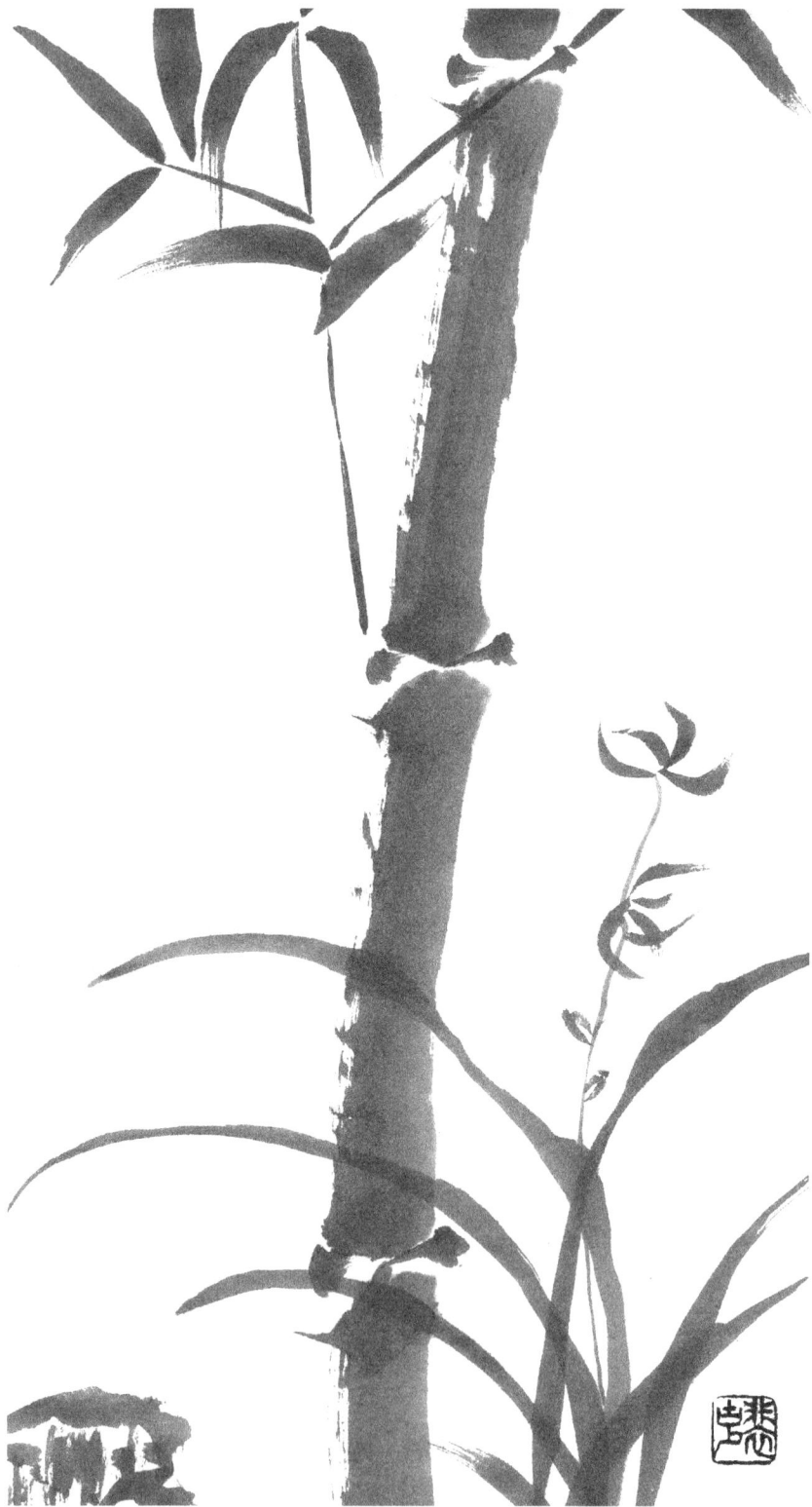

# CHAPTER TWENTY-THREE

An hour after Liu and Pei Ke left Huo's home, they were ambushed. The two attackers rushed from the outcroppings alongside the road. They ignored Pei Ke and charged at Liu.

From the corner of his eye, Liu saw the attack coming from the right. At first, he thought there was only one. Immediately he went into the Dragon Palm posture of Pa Kua Chang and started to walk a circle around the linear attack. The opponent recognized the movement and changed the angle of attack to counter Liu's maneuver. The attacker's fist made contact with Liu's right arm as Liu blocked the attack. Suddenly, Pei Ke screamed and Liu sighed inwardly. He had no choice in what he needed to do next. He had to protect Pei Ke.

He made a few quick foot adjustments and switched from Pa Kua Chang to Hsing-Yi Chuan. He further closed the short distance to the attacker and used a modified version of the Tiger posture of Hsing-Yi Chuan. Normally, both his hands would be slightly apart as he made contact, but he placed his left hand on top of his right hand, concentrating the force of the move.

As his palms made contact with the attacker's chest, Liu opened his shoulders slightly so the Qi could flow from the earth, through his upper back, and then to his hands. The first sound was the exhalation of air from the opponent's chest, followed by the sound of the sternum and ribs breaking. The attacker's heart stopped instantly as the Qi penetrated directly to the spine and went up to the head and down to the earth. Blood started dripping from the man's mouth. His eyes rolled backward and upward as he collapsed.

Liu turned to see the source of Pei Ke's scream. Seeing the other man, he reverted back to the Dragon Palm of Pa Kua Chang and began walking the circle, this time counter clockwise. He moved fast but not fast enough to avoid the six-inch cut from a sword that slashed the area of his left scapula. Liu felt the pain almost instantly. He knew from the angle of attack that the sword sliced downward, away from his body. He closed the distance as blood stained his shirt.

He blocked an attempted sword thrust. His right hand went directly to the man's throat. He positioned his fingers alongside the throat protrusion and squeezed so that his fingers encircled the opponents Adam's apple. When his fingers met, they penetrated the skin. Blood squirted out through both sides of the opponent's throat. Liu pulled forward and downward and the attacker collapsed to the ground gasping for air. The assailant thrashed on the ground for a few seconds and then lay still. Liu knew it was a cruel death, but he had no choice. He was wounded and didn't know if there were more attackers.

"Master, are you all right?" Pei Ke quickly came to Liu's side.

"Is that all of them?" Liu said. "Did you see any more?"

"No, Master," Pei Ke said, looking around anyway. "Are you alright?"

"Yes, in my old age I am getting slow. He should never have gotten that close."

"But Master, you're hurt."

"Yes. I am cut on my upper back. I will need your help to stop the bleeding. In my pack there is some Yun Nan Bai Yao. Please get it for me."

"What does it look like?"

"It is wrapped in paper. The name is on the paper. Be careful not to spill the powder."

Pei Ke found the paper packet and carefully put it aside.

"Help me take off my shirt," Liu said.

Pei Ke had only once seen Liu without a shirt. For an old man, his skin was taut and the muscles well-defined. Pei Ke examined the area where the sword had cut. Thankfully, it was superficial and not life-threatening.

"Pei Ke, open the paper packet and sprinkle the powder on the cut. This will stop the bleeding so that the healing process can start."

"Master, how much do I put on?"

"Just enough to cover the cut. Do not waste it on the surrounding area. You may have to do it more than once to stop the bleeding."

As Pei Ke carefully applied the herb to Liu's wound, he thought about the dead men. Why had they attacked Liu? They had been attacked so many times during their journey that it was becoming more and more clear that somebody wanted the Master dead. He could not imagine who and the thought scared him.

"Master, most of the bleeding has stopped."

"Put a little more of the herb on the areas that are still bleeding."

"Yes, Master."

After a few minutes, Pei Ke saw that the bleeding had completely stopped. He touched Liu's skin and felt the softness of the skin, but the hardness of the muscles. He touched his own skin and felt the difference. His skin was soft and his muscles were hard, but not as hard as Liu's.

"Master, what should we do with these bodies?" He tried not to look at the man whose throat Liu had ripped out, but he could not avoid it. "Should we take them someplace or just leave them as we did the last time."

"Help me with my shirt."

Pei Ke helped Liu with his shirt. The older man showed no outward indication of any pain, but he was careful so that the wound would not reopen.

"Let's go," said Liu.

"Master, do you want to take this sword in case we need to defend ourselves again?" Pei Ke gestured to the weapon lying beside the dead man.

Liu did not answer the question and never looked back as the two of them continued on their journey north. Pei Ke's mind was full of questions, but he felt it was inappropriate to bother his master then. Once again, his master and teacher had proven himself in close combat, and once again he felt helpless. This weighed heavily on him. He wanted to follow in his teacher's footsteps and be a great martial arts master, even if it meant being poor the rest of his life. He marveled at how calm Liu had been during and after the altercation. Pei Ke felt the anxiety in his own body and did not know how to calm himself. He was shaking and he wished for that inner strength he saw in Liu.

Pei Ke looked back where the two dead men had fallen, but they were no longer there. At first, he thought they were too far away from the scene, but when he could still see the narrowing of the rock outcropping, he knew he was looking at the right place. He was also sure that Liu had killed the two men. There was no way they could have survived the injuries they sustained, and so they could not have fled. Someone must have moved the bodies, which meant there were more of them, and that they were still being followed.

"Master, the two bodies are gone."

"Yes, those two weren't alone. I am sure that soon, we will meet up with the rest of them. I think we are safe for today, but let's hurry and get to our next destination before nightfall."

# CHAPTER TWENTY-FOUR

"Master, we've been traveling for sixteen days and each night, we've stopped at an interesting place. Are we doing so again tonight?"

"We will be visiting Wei Ken De, one of my first students. He studied Pa Kua Chang and Hsing-Yi Chuan and now lives in a small community north of here."

"Does he teach?"

"Yes. He teaches a small group of students, but he is very selective in whom he accepts. He learned other martial arts before studying with me and teaches his students a combination of what I taught him and what he had learned."

"Did he study with you at the temple? I don't remember ever seeing him."

Liu shook his head.

"He is one of my 'inner door' students: he learned privately. Before I moved to the temple, he would visit me, but later, after I began living in the temple, he would return often for instruction. He was a gifted, intuitive student. I seldom had to correct him."

"He must be talented."

"Yes, he is brilliant, and his desire to excel shows in his martial arts and in his work. He is also successful in business. Many people hold him in high respect. He is consistent and tenacious, yet he is willing to listen and learn without asking too many questions. I teach him because of his dedication and his ability. Some students have ability but no loyalty, and others have loyalty but no ability. He has both." He looked at Pei Ke firmly.

"Loyalty is very important," he said. "Do not forget that. Someday you will have the opportunity to teach. You do not want to teach your students your martial art treasures only to find that they do not honor you as their teacher. Sooner or later, these students will leave to teach on their own. They will attract students with their ability and words, but fail for one reason or another to fully disclose you as their teacher. It is an error of omission on their part."

Pei Ke nodded, then thoughtfully said, "If you taught Wei Ken De and now you are teaching me, than Wei Ken De and I are martial art brothers."

"Yes, but he is senior to you, so you must show him the necessary respect. He can help you if you need instruction if I am not available."

"Where are all your other students?"

"Over the years many students have studied from me. They have come…"

Liu paused and looked at Pei Ke, but then said no more.

They had been walking for about an hour when Liu suddenly stopped and looked into the distance. Pei Ke found it strange that Liu would stare for a couple of seconds and then continue walking. It began to make him uncomfortable. When he'd look in the same direction, he saw nothing, but he remembered the vanishing bodies of the day before and Liu's warning that they were still being followed. He had no idea what Liu had done to make him such a target, but he began to feel as though they were being watched by sinister eyes.

Then, as the road made a sharp turn, Liu suddenly grabbed Pei Ke's shirt and pulled him off the road into the forest, motioning for him to follow and be quiet. They went thirty feet into the woods, just enough to be hidden, but not so far to prevent them from seeing anyone passing on the road.

Ten minutes went by and they saw no one. Pei Ke was overwhelmed with questions, but he kept quiet. Ten minutes turned into twenty minutes and then thirty, until at last Liu rose and they walked back to the road.

"Master, are they still there?"

"Yes, at least one and maybe two people are still following us. I wanted to see who they were, but they obviously did not want to be seen."

Pei Ke looked around nervously. The terrain made it unlikely that anyone had passed them by any means other than the road, which meant the villains were still behind them.

"Who are these people?" he asked desperately.

"Not our friends, obviously," Liu said.

"Does all this have anything to do with that letter you received? Why would anyone want to hurt you?" This was the first time he had ever directly talked to his master about the contents of the letter and when Liu looked at him, he wondered if he had made a mistake in doing so.

"There is nothing in the letter that directly suggests a connection between its contents and our adventures," Liu said finally. "But there are many indirect hints. I do not know what they want with me, but I will know soon. Come. We have many miles to travel still. If those who follow us decide to try their skill against me, they will learn what their friends did."

"Yes, Master," Pei Ke said. Occasionally, during the next two hours, he would scan the surrounding countryside, though he didn't know what he was looking for.

"We are almost there," Liu said at last and Pei Ke felt the tension in his shoulders finally begin to relax. "We made good time despite that little distraction. We will be at my student's house before the sun goes down."

Pei Ke could see a village up ahead as they came over a small rise. He thought that a community in the middle of this rough terrain would be very small, maybe ten or fifteen houses, but there were a couple hundred houses. It seemed peaceful and lush, far different than what they encountered previously in the evil area.

Liu guided them down one street and then another. Once again, he led them in circles and Pei Ke was grateful for it. Occasionally, his master would stop and wait and listen. He would look in all directions, as if he expected to see someone, and then they would continue. Each time, Pei Ke wanted to ask what he had heard, or seen, but he knew better than to do so.

Each street looked like the one before, and as in other villages they had passed through, the walls along the streets were covered with hundreds of little pieces of paper with every imaginable notice. Some advertised services while others gave blessings to the masses. They passed by what appeared to be the local magistrate's office. A short distance later, they came to an inconspicuous wall with a faded red door. Nothing about it suggested who might live there. Liu knocked on the door and then pulled the braided rope, which rang a bell inside the house. Pei Ke heard the opening and closing of a door.

"Who is there?" asked the voice on the other side of the door.

"I am Liu Bin. Is Wei Ken De here?"

A bolt slid silently to one side, and a small peephole opened and darkened. Then, the door quickly swung open and a tall, thin man with a penciled mustache and a scar on his left cheek stood in the doorway. A crooked smile lit up his face.

"Master, please come in! What a pleasant surprise. Come in. Come in."

"I know that I am unexpected," Liu said. "Is it an inconvenience for us to be here?"

"Of course not. The master has given me standing orders to make you welcome whether or not they are here. This home is always open to you."

Liu and Pei Ke walked into the expansive outer courtyard. Pei Ke saw a well-manicured and pleasant scene, much different from what he had seen on the outside. They had moved from one lifestyle to another by walking through a portal. As they walked toward the house, he saw beautiful plants arranged into a pleasing harmony, which reminded him of the peacefulness he felt in both the Taoist and Buddhist temples they had visited. From the look of the plants and the way they were being cultivated, he knew this was an herb garden. To the right were many pots with different flowers. To his left were large pots that he suspected contained goldfish.

Pei Ke could see chimes dangling from one corner of the roof. He knew the chimes were there to ward off any evil spirits lurking about. He sighed inwardly in relief. After their experience in the evil village, Pei Ke had been having nightmares about evil spirits. In his dreams the spirits were following him wherever he went. Knowing that they were actually being followed made him uneasy. He found comfort in the chimes that warded off evil spirits. This house was well protected.

As they approached the front door, it opened as if by some unseen command and a second servant greeted Liu.

"Master Liu, have you eaten?" this second servant asked.

The man did not have a bit of fat on his body and Pei Ke noticed that he walked similarly to Liu, as though he were rooted to the ground but his steps were somehow light and unhindered by any resistance. Pei Ke thought he would have to ask his master about this man when he had a chance. For now, he just watched and followed.

"No," Liu responded. "We have been traveling all day, and we are tired and hungry." He introduced Pei Ke and they entered the house, following the servant to a sitting area.

"I will let my Master know you are here," the servant said. "Please, have a seat. He will be happy you have come again. I will see to your accommodations for the evening and make sure the cook knows to add two more for dinner."

Liu motioned for Pei Ke to sit down while he walked around the room. Pei Ke thought the room was one of the most beautifully decorated he had ever seen. The house was even more ornate than the living quarters at the teahouse. He thought it odd how many rich people his master knew. He took comfort knowing that at least one of Liu's students was wealthy.

After a few moments, Pei Ke heard the quick steps of someone walking down the hallway. As he looked up, he saw a tall thin man enter the room and bow in deep respect to Liu.

"Master, this is such a surprise!" the man who was clearly Wei Ken De said. "You will of course eat and stay the night with us."

Liu introduced Pei Ke who bowed in respect to Liu's senior student. As their eyes met, Pei Ke immediately knew where his place was in the hierarchy of Liu's students. The intenseness of the man's eyes took Pei Ke by surprise. Pei Ke felt the man's energy. He needed to remember his place, but he also wondered what things Liu had taught this man. Pei Ke hoped there would be time to befriend Wei Ken De before they left.

"Master, please have a seat. Your visit is a pleasant surprise. Just the other day, I mentioned to my daughter that we needed to spend some time with you. Will you be staying long with us?"

"No," Liu said. "Only for one night. There is trouble at my home."

Wei Ken De's eyebrow lifted in concern.

"Trouble?"

Liu nodded.

"I received a note, supposedly from my brother, requesting that I return home as soon as possible."

"That is concerning," Wei Ken De said, though it was clear from his tone that he suspected more was coming.

"The handwriting was not my brother's," Liu said. "We have been followed ever since we left the temple. We lost them here in the city streets. I am confident they did not follow us to your house, but they clearly know where I am going. They will probably wait on the outskirts of the village. I do not know what I will find when I arrive home. My intuition tells me that there is trouble."

If Pei Ke's initial introduction to Wei Ken De had not been enough to show him his place, listening to the two men talk would have. Not only was Liu willing to speak openly of the contents of the letter and his personal concerns, which he had clearly kept from Pei Ke, it was clear that Liu valued Wei Ken De's opinion. They spoke almost as equals.

Pei Ke listened as his master explained the events of their journey and found it refreshing to hear things from his master's point of view. Each attack was nothing more than an occurrence, an indication more of some impending larger confrontation. Pei Ke wondered at his master's ability to take such things in stride and felt fortunate that he was Liu's student.

"Is there something I can do to help?" asked Wei Ken De when the story was finished.

"Yes," Liu said. "You are helping us already by putting us up for the evening."

"Shall I go with you?" Wei Ken De asked. "I can be of help if there is trouble." Pei Ke thought the senior student had glanced at him and was glad that Liu had downplayed Pei Ke's own inefficacy during his narrative, though he suspected Wei Ken De knew.

"No, it is best you remain here with your daughter. There is little you can do, and I do not want you to be drawn into whatever is ahead."

Wei Ken De turned to Pei Ke and was about to say something, but Liu spoke again.

"There is another thing you can do for me. Are you still training your servant in martial arts?"

"Yes," Wei Ken De said. "I teach him when I teach my daughter." He noticed Pei Ke's look of surprise and smiled faintly.

"It is not customary to train servants," Liu said, answering the unspoken question, "but in some cases of unswerving loyalty, it is appropriate. You remember what I said of loyalty?" Liu looked directly at Pei Ke.

"Yes, Master," Pei Ke said.

"How good is the man?" Liu said, returning his attention to Wei Ken De.

"He is fair. Why?"

"Can he explore the area to see if he could learn anything about those men who are following us? Maybe they have made inquiries about a place to stay. It would be helpful to know where and when to expect them again."

"Yes, it will be done. Is there anything else?"

"No, though I would like to see your daughter. I have not seen her for some time."

"I will go and let her know you are here. I want to give my servant some instructions and check on our meal and your sleeping arrangements for the evening."

As Wei Ken De stood up he looked directly at Pei Ke, and once again Pei Ke felt a power or force within this man.

After the door closed, Pei Ke turned to Liu. "How long has Wei Ken De been studying with you?"

"Is that important?" Liu answered.

"No, Master. Please forgive my bad manners."

A long silence followed before Liu spoke.

"Wei Ken De has been studying with me for many years. For the first few years, he would come in the mornings and practice for a couple of hours. Later, when his endurance and strength increased, he would practice twice a day. The rest of the time, he worked in one of the local shops.

"He chose to practice martial arts because he loved the art. His father disapproved of him wasting his time practicing, but Wei Ken De felt that he needed to learn martial arts at that juncture in his life. His father was quite well to do and sometimes sent him a little money to support his meager existence. That was over twenty years ago. He is still practicing and learning. He now has his own students…"

The door opened slowly and they turned to see who had entered the room.

To Pei Ke, she was the most beautiful woman he had ever seen. He wondered if anyone had heard him gasp. Her complexion was radiant with a special quality that made one stare and then become embarrassed for staring. Pei Ke was very familiar with embarrassment, but this was different than anything he had ever felt. He was suddenly aware of every flaw he had and had the sinking feeling that she did as well.

"Master Liu, Father said you were here." Pei Ke found a renewal of his embarrassment. "I could not believe it! It has been so long since you have honored this house with your presence."

The girl made a perfect bow of respect to Liu and Liu acknowledged the bow, smiling.

"Mei Li, this is Pei Ke. He is studying and traveling with me."

Mei Li looked at Pei Ke and bowed. He didn't know what to do. Awkwardly, he returned the bow.

"Master, how long will you stay?" she said. "My father keeps telling me stories about you. I have so many questions to ask."

Before Liu could answer, the door opened and Wei Ken De returned.

"Wei Ken De, I would like to have a word with you in private before we eat," Liu said. "It will only take a few minutes."

Wei Ken De turned to his daughter."Would you be so kind as to take Pei Ke and show him around for a few minutes? I will call for both of you when we are done."

At the thought of being alone with this beautiful girl, Pei Ke nearly panicked, but he realized that she was probably as nervous as he was. It was highly unusual for a daughter to be left with an unknown man, though she clearly had the confidence and poise to handle it well. They began to walk and she spoke eloquently of various scrolls or architectural points. After a few minutes, his natural curiosity began to assert itself and replace his nerves.

"You have a very nice home," he finally said. "Have you lived here all your life?"

"Yes. This house belonged to my grandfather and my parents have lived here since before I was born. When my grandparents passed away, my father inherited the house. I was born sometime after that. "Her eyes became distant and she sighed.

"I never met my grandparents," she said, "and my mother passed away a few years ago. Now, it is just my father, me, and the servants. Actually, my mother died three years ago next month, with both of us at her side."

"I am sorry," Pei Ke said. He wanted to comfort her. Clearly, speaking of her mother made her sad, but he was lost for words. He wanted to console her, but felt awkward. He again noticed how beautiful she was. He had never seen anyone with such beauty.

"Thank you," she said. For a fleeting moment, she looked into his eyes and he thought maybe she understood what he wanted to say but could not. Then, she diverted her gaze and looked downward modestly.

Pei Ke instantly felt weak. Feelings unlike anything he had experienced washed over him. He searched for something to say.

"Do you have any brothers and sisters?" asked Mei Li.

"Yes," he said, grateful to be talking about something familiar. "I have a brother and a sister. My brother and his wife live by the temple where Master Liu stays. My sister lives with her husband. And you?" He suddenly became nervous that she had lost siblings as well as a mother. He followed her across the patterned wood floors that were strewn with woven rugs.

"No," said Mei Li. "Mother did not have any more children after me. Of course, I got all the attention, but it would have been nice to have other siblings. I now try to help my father by running the house. I know I cannot replace my mother, but I try to help him as much as possible."

As Mei Li talked, Pei Ke took in as much as possible of what she was saying as well as what she was not saying. Her beauty captivated him. She was modestly dressed but unknowingly sensual in her mannerisms. Her beautiful eyes and smile enhanced her tall, womanly appearance.

As they walked down a long hallway, Pei Ke again noticed scrolls and the ornate trappings of the house. Mei Li opened a door and motioned for him to enter. It was a large room with chairs along the walls, but with no other furniture except an altar. Pei Ke smelled the lingering odor of burnt incense. Behind the altar was a scroll with Liu's name written in big characters and on the far wall, a well-secured door appeared to lead to the outside. Various weapons were hung neatly on the walls. Two well-worn circles lay in the center of the floor. Pei Ke instantly understood the significance of the circles.

They were silent for a moment, and then Pei Ke said, "Do you practice martial arts."

"Yes," she said. "I started training at the age of six. Of course, when I was very young, I mostly learned strength building exercises. As I grew older Father began teaching me Hsing-Yi Chuan and I have been practicing it ever since."

Pei Ke realized Mei Li had been studying martial arts longer than he had. He tried to imagine her practicing Hsing-Yi Chuan. She was very feminine and Hsing-Yi Chuan was not feminine at all. He imagined that she must be very accomplished by now.

"Master Liu said you were his student," she asked.

"Yes, I study with him in the mornings on the mountain next to the temple."

"You are very lucky. I am happy to study from my father, but it is truly an honor to study from Master Liu. Father indicates that he is very selective and has turned down many potential students. He must see a special quality in you."

There was something in the way she said it, as though there was some deeper significance to her words, but he couldn't imagine what that significance was.

"Yes," he said, hoping he wasn't blushing. "I am fortunate to have Master Liu as my teacher. He is a master in so many fields. Ultimately, I would like to be a doctor and treat patients with acupuncture and herbs, though I also want to be a martial artist like Master Liu and your father. You are fortunate you have your father to instruct you all the time. I only get to see Master Liu in the mornings when we practice. He is teaching me Hsing-Yi Chuan as well, though recently he started teaching me Pa Kua Chang. I like them both. I especially like when Master Liu makes comparisons between the two arts."

"I don't know Pa Kua Chang," said Mei Li, "though, I've seen my father practice it and teach it countless times. I find that comparing Hsing-Yi and Pa Kua is like comparing the concepts of Yin and Yang: it is not a true comparison. Hsing-Yi is very linear and somewhat masculine. The movements of Pa Kua seem to be circular and smooth and in some cases very feminine. I would imagine that you like Hsing-Yi because it is harder and more linear."

Pei Ke thought about it, though he was distracted by the way she bit her lower lip when she was thinking.

"I like your masculine-feminine comparison with these two martial arts," he said. "I have thought the same thing before, though I do not prefer one over the other. Each works in the proper context, and so I like them differently at different times. Hsing-Yi Chuan is more suited for power and attacking, and Pa Kua Chang is better for finesse and dissolving an attack. It is nice to know both of them, so one can shift between appropriate styles as necessary."

He thought of Liu and the various mêlées in which he had recently seen him. He had no trouble shifting between styles. Pei Ke hoped he sounded like his master a little when he spoke of it and he realized that it had become easy to talk with Mei Li.

She was certainly not the first female who had made him feel embarrassed or nervous. There were many times before when he felt uncomfortable with women of his own age. He did not quite understand them, and he never knew what to say. On those occasions when he did say something, he often felt like it was inappropriate somehow, and they would invariably giggle or laugh. He was never sure if they were laughing at him or because they too were nervous, but he was sure the uncertainty could not be a good thing when it came to courting.

Before his parents passed away, they had often suggested girls they thought would be suitable wives for him. He had never been interested in their suggestions. He found the women either unattractive or dull witted. He wanted someone he could talk with, someone whose common interests forged a bond between them, and he realized that Mei Li so far seemed to fulfill all these criteria.

He knew his wishes were totally contrary to the prevailing customs, but that didn't matter to him. It was his life, and he liked to think he was someone who walked a separate path. Maybe that was why he was so attracted to Liu Bin: Liu walked his own path.

He thought suddenly of Master's repeated warnings that his path was lonely and simultaneously, he wondered what path Mei Li was taking. He thought again how beautiful she was and how wonderful he felt for the first time in his life. He instinctively turned to look at her and saw that she was looking at him with a warm smile. His heart skipped a beat as he turned his head away.

———————

Liu and Wei Ken De were seated across from each other. Wei Ken De waited for his teacher to start the conversation.

"Pei Ke has been studying with me for some time now," said Liu. "He seems to have both the talent and loyalty needed to be a good student. I may send him to you for further training. Whatever you feel appropriate to teach him will be fine with me. I have modified some of the moves I taught you to suit him because of his stature."

He paused, but Wei Ken De said nothing, waiting. Liu smiled to himself. The man really was a great student.

"Do you remember what I told you years ago?" he said. "Do not teach anyone anything unless they are ready to learn."

Again, he paused. After a respectful minute, Wei Ken De finally broke the silence.

"Master, I have studied with you for many years. If you wish for me to train Pei Ke, then of course I will do so. You are like a father to me."

Liu nodded. Now it was his turn to wait.

"Master," Wei Ken De said. "I am grateful you have come. I have no one to turn to when I have questions."

"If you would like to ask questions, please do so. Neither one of us knows when our paths will cross again. Dispense with the formality and ask."

"I guess it is really a combination of questions and insight. It is nice to be able to ask you questions."

"Indeed," Liu smiled. He waved his hand, indicating for Wei Ken De to proceed.

"You have mentioned before that in the internal martial arts, intention is a vital component. I have always understood the words, but never understood the meaning, until now. I think I finally understand.

"As you have so eloquently stated before, we are a system of energy within a system. If we can make our own system healthy and function at its optimum, then we can have an influence over other human systems.

"Collectively, the people on earth make another system, thus we are a system within a system. Since we are systems, we radiate energy and this energy can affect the energy of nearby systems. That is why we can will something to happen, or anticipate when someone is going to attack, or will our energy to travel from our back to our hand, like when we use Fa Jing. We sense the energy of the system and tap into that energy."

"You are correct," said Liu. "Though, there is more to it."

"Master, I assume that my system can function well or poorly depending on how I take care of the system. My question is, why do some students progress in the development of their systems and others do not?"

"There are many factors," said Liu. "First, their systems can be affected by a genetic or hereditary factor. Intelligent students come from intelligent parents. Now that you have been teaching, you realize that some people have ability and some do not. This applies to the physical, mental, emotional, and spiritual aspects of our lives.

"Second, their systems can be affected by their development since birth, and that is where parents are the primary influence on development. The third factor is the competence of the teacher and the ability to explain the dynamics of energy. This assumes the teacher knows what he is talking about. Many teachers claim to know martial arts and Qi Gong, but really do not."

"Master, from a physical aspect, what will help move the Qi in my body?" asked Wei Ken De.

"As you know, each time that you came for instruction I took care to ensure that there was proper alignment of your body, that your head was suspended from above, and your breathing was correct. This was all designed to make sure that the energy was not blocked by tense muscles and closed joints. The opening of the joints is important. That is why stretching is so important in the development of Qi; it opens the joints."

He continued to answer Wei Ken De's questions until the servant announced their meal. Liu enjoyed talking with his old students. Each of them had taken a different course in life, but he felt connected to each of them and gained strength from that connection. He realized that he even felt that connection with Pei Ke, as young as he was. He was glad the boy was with him. For what was coming, he would need all the strength he could gather.

––––––––––

The dinner was sumptuous. The cook outdid himself in providing the correct amount of Yin vegetables and Yang vegetables designed to balance and enhance energy. Pei Ke sat across from Mei Li at the table. It was customary for women to eat by themselves when male guests were present, but Mei Li's father wanted her to be part of his life. Pei Ke and Mei Li were silent as Liu and Wei Ken De shared experiences since their last meeting.

Pei Ke tried to follow the conversation, but was deep in thought about Mei Li. The more he thought about her, the more he was attracted to her beauty and poise. It seemed odd to him that he would feel thus after only their first meeting, but he could not avoid the fact that she would make a perfect wife. She could run the house and he could work. The only problem was that he was poorer than a temple mouse, and she came from an educated and well-to-do family. He wondered if there ever would be a chance for him to court her. He noticed that she glanced in his direction from time to time. This was not unnoticed by Liu and Wei Ken De.

"Pei Ke."

He was deep in thought when his name was spoken.

"Yes," Pei Ke said, somewhat startled.

"I understand from Master Liu that you are studying martial arts."

"Yes," said Pei Ke. "Master Liu has been kind enough to teach me, but I am only a beginner in these arts. I want to learn everything that I can learn."

"I would be interested in hearing what he has been teaching you, "Wei Ken De said and Pei Ke nodded as respectfully as he could.

"Master, are you full?" asked Wei Ken De, suddenly turning his attention back to Liu. "Is there anything else you need?"

"No," said Liu. "The meal was superb."

"Father," Mei Li said. "While you and Pei Ke talk, I would like to show Master Liu some of our new paintings."

"Of course," Wei Ken De said.

Liu and Mei Li got up from the table leaving Pei Ke at the mercy of Wei Ken De's questioning.

———————

"Master," Mei Li said when they had entered a private room, "May I talk to you about a minor problem I've been having? I'm a little embarrassed, because it is a female problem, and I don't want you to feel uncomfortable."

Liu smiled.

"I treat both men and women. I do not think of a personal conversation as anything other than an opportunity to help, so please do not feel uncomfortable. You are of age, so of course, anything that you share with me will be held in confidence."

"Thank you, Master. All my girlfriends have started their monthly period, but I have not. When mother was alive, she told me it would come soon and not to worry. My friends are talking about marriage and having children, but unless I have a period, I will not have children."

"Has your father had any discussions with other families about a potential husband for you?"

"He has had discussions, but I don't think he has anyone in mind. He has extremely high standards and there are many young men my age and older that he does not really like."

"Have you met any nice young men?"

"No. Well, maybe yes."

Liu paused and then smiled and looked her directly in the eyes.

"You need to meet a nice young man who shares your same interests. That way you will have something in common and something to share the rest of your lives."

"Master, do you know of someone my father would approve?"

"Perhaps, but you are still young. Enjoy life while you are young. Now, let me ask you a few questions about your health issues. Did your mother indicate when she started to menstruate?"

"Yes, I asked her and she said she also started late, but she did not tell me the exact age."

"Did your mother have severe menstrual cramps?"

"Yes. Sometimes they were minimal, but there were also times when she had to take some herbs. The herbs really helped as they eased the pain considerably. Do you know what herbs she was taking?"

"I don't know what her signs and symptoms were or the feeling of her pulses. It could have been a number of different combinations. Do you have any other health issues?"

"Only some acne. It only lasts a few days, and then goes away."

"How long before the acne returns?"

"It comes back periodically. It isn't much of a concern."

"Do you have breast tenderness at any time?"

"Yes." She paused, then asked, "Are there any acupuncture points to help with that problem?"

"Yes. There are acupuncture points that will help with this problem."

"Master, do you know these points?"

"Yes, of course." said Liu. "Do you have any problems with urination or bowel movements?"

"No. When I was very young I had some problems, but mother gave me some herbs and that solved the problem."

"Do you have any aches, pains, or sore joints anywhere in your body?"

"Yes, my lower back hurts quite often. I assume it comes from practicing martial arts. My knees ache also."

"How are you feeling emotionally? Do you have any episodes of fear or depression?"

"Often I feel tired mentally and sometimes I am depressed. I think of my mother often and really miss her."

"Do you like to eat or drink cold things?"

"Yes, I do like to drink cold things. I know I am not supposed to have anything cold, but I do enjoy it often. Sometimes I feel cold inside."

"Do you eat regular meals?"

"Yes, I eat regular meals. We eat at almost the same time each day."

"Do you eat meat?"

"No, Master, we do not eat meat. We are vegetarians like you."

"Do you eat fish?"

"No, it is very difficult to get fish in this part of the country. People get fish from the rivers, but we do not have fish."

"Do you eat eggs?"

"No."

"Have you ever eaten meat, fish, or eggs?"

"We are Buddhist, as you know, and we want to be in harmony with nature. Why do you ask the question?"

"There is a strong correlation between body fat and a woman's menstruation. You are in rigorous martial arts training. I know your father is training you hard and you should be thankful he takes an interest in your martial arts development. Your mother and father are both thin. You are very thin and tall. Young women who exercise a lot and are thin have less body fat, which may delay the onset of menses. Eating a little meat and fish will help your body build up a little fat and strengthen itself. Your constitution will then be stronger and able to support the menstrual cycle."

"So I should eat a little meat or fish to help get my period started?"

"It is more complex than that. We need to find out about your energy patterns and see if you have any disharmonies. Do you have other health issues?"

"Master, my lungs feel tight most of the time."

"Do you cough often?"

"Sometimes I cough for no reason at all."

"Do you cough anything up?"

"No, but it feels like there is a band around my chest. The tightness varies throughout the year. When I practice regularly I don't have the problem."

Liu felt her pulses, paying particular attention on the lung pulse.

"There are some acupuncture points we can use to help with this problem."

"Where are the points located?" asked Mei Li.

"If you use Gong Sun on the Yin surface of the foot and Nei Guan on the Yin surface of the arm in combination with special points in the ear, the lungs will expand and you will be able to breathe more deeply. Actually, we use nine needles in the ear. These points in the ear are very effective for people who have been subjected to a lot of dust, or have inhaled a lot of smoke for a long time. It is interesting how these ear points affect the lungs. Each time you insert a needle, the patient will feel a different part of his lungs relaxing and opening up. If you take a piece of rice paper and draw a pair of lungs on the paper, and then insert needles one at a time into these special points in the ear, the patient will be able to mark on the paper exactly where the lungs are opening. You will be able to see a pattern developing. Now, I need to feel your pulses once more. They will tell me about the energy in your body and what is the correct method for treating you."

Again, Liu felt the pulses on both her right and left wrists. He took his time, first placing his middle finger on the middle pulse, then the index finger on the wrist pulse, and finally his ring finger on the last pulse. He pressed each pulse separately, feeling for a superficial pulse and a deep pulse. Each pulse told him a specific thing about the energy flow in Mei Li's body.

As he was feeling the throbbing of her heart pulse, he noticed that she became distracted and her eyes became distant. Suddenly, he felt a change in the pulse rate on the heart meridian and a change in the quality of the pulse. He also noticed a slight smile forming on Mei Li's face. He had felt this change before when treating other young women. Affairs of the heart were interesting, he thought to himself. He had never allowed himself to become involved with the ways of the heart. His bliss was totally within himself, but he understood he was unusual and that others had their own paths to follow.

"Master, how long has Pei Ke been studying with you?"

"A few years."

"Does his astrological sign make him a good candidate to be a martial artist and doctor?"

"Being a monkey, he is very resourceful."

Mei Li inwardly smiled realizing that Pei Ke's astrological sign was compatible with hers.

Liu next looked at Mei Li's tongue checking for any abnormalities that would give him a clue as to why she had not yet started her period. He noticed her tongue was a little pale—a little too pale for someone who was an athlete. She had no substantial white or yellow coating on the tongue. Next, he felt her abdomen for any masses or lumps, but did not find anything of concern.

"When a young woman has not had her first period, it can be due to several factors: blood deficiency, kidney deficiency, or coldness in the uterus. In your situation, I think that the intense exercise, low body fat, vegetarian diet, your physique, lower back and knee pain, your emotions associated with your mother's death, and the tendency to drink cold things combine to suggest kidney deficiency and blood deficiency. This is not in itself a serious problem. It can be corrected by slightly changing your diet to include some meat and taking some herbs. I will write an herbal prescription for you before I leave. It is important to drink the herbal concoction while it is very warm. Warm herbs have a better effect on your body. You have just had a very full meal. It would not be appropriate to do acupuncture now. If there is time we will do it later. Be sure and go to the herbalist in the morning."

Liu went on to explain more of the dynamics of her situation, pointing out some of the important factors concerning the changes in her body she needed to be aware of while she was taking the herbs.

————————

While Liu and Mei Li were talking, Pei Ke and Wei Ken De were having what Pei Ke thought was a one-sided conversation.

"Master Liu and I have not yet had a chance to have a good conversation," Wei Ken De said. "We will probably have an opportunity to visit later this evening. I have known Master Liu and his family for many years. I remember when I first met him. I was in awe with how powerful he looked. Because of my father, Liu readily accepted me as a student. His instruction changed my whole life. I don't think I could ever find a more knowledgeable person. It is quite an honor to be one of his students. You are very fortunate."

"I do feel fortunate to study with him. What has he taught you over the years?"

Wei Ken De ignored the question. "How did you meet Master Liu?"

"I saw him practicing his art early one morning as I was climbing the mountain. I watched from a distance for a number of days. One day I went to watch him and he was not there. I waited for a few minutes. When I turned to leave, he was behind me. At first, I thought he would be angry and think I was spying on him or trying to steal his secrets. Instead he invited me to practice with him. I was more apprehensive than nervous. He assured me there was no problem. I started to practice, and he taught me more each time I went to visit."

"What has he taught you?"

"I have learned some Qi Gong, Hsing-Yi Chuan, and Pa Kua Chang."

"Master Liu knows many different martial art forms. Have you learned all the forms?"

"No, not yet, but he has taught me quite a bit."

"How long have you been studying with him?"

"About two years. I want to learn everything he knows, including martial arts, medicine, calligraphy, and painting."

"It will take you many years to learn. Do you have all that time to spend with him?"

"I work, but I have many hours to practice and study."

"You seem dedicated to what you are doing. Do you ever get tired of practicing?"

"No. I enjoy every bit of it."

As Wei Ken De continued to ask questions, Pei Ke wondered why Liu's senior student was so curious. He felt as though Wei Ken De was searching for some information.

"Why do you want to become a doctor? It is a very important and demanding profession. Do you think you can handle the responsibility?"

"I have seen Master Liu treat patients. I know it will take many years for me to learn correctly. He has so much to teach and I am willing to learn. Hopefully, when I finish studying, I will be ready to assume the responsibility that comes with the profession."

"Master Liu has had many teachers over the years. To study from these teachers, he had to travel to different parts of the country. He is getting old and may not be around for you to finish your training. "Wei Ken De spoke as if he were reading from a list of questions he had prepared earlier in the day.

"Right now, he is able and willing to teach me. I need to take advantage of his kindness and learn as much as possible from him."

Pei Ke knew his time with Liu might be short, but the reality of this thought had not materialized until he said it aloud. More than ever, he needed to focus all his efforts on what he was doing and not become distracted. He felt this trip had helped to renew his devotion.

"Have you thought about settling down and taking over your father's business?" Wei Ken De asked.

"My parents have passed away. Of course, my father would have liked me to follow in his footsteps, but I wanted to do something else with my life. It is almost impossible for someone like me to move from my low level of existence to a position of honor and dignity. I was not born into a wealthy family, nor did my father have any connections with anyone of influence. Studying with Master Liu is one way for me and my future children to gain status and wealth."

Pei Ke thought Wei Ken De smiled, but when he looked again, the man's lips were as flat as ever.

"You may want to resolve a contradiction existing in your statements," the older man said. "If you want to be like Master Liu, you will have to actually be like Master Liu. He has no money and no aspirations to acquire money. If you have a family, how would you be able to support them?"

"I have not thought much about having a family or a wife. "An image of Mei Li flashed through his mind. "I need to study and train. I am still very young. A wife and family can come later."

———————

That night, Liu Bin answered all the questions Wei Ken De had wanted to ask him. Liu knew the level and quality of questions was indicative of the level of training and understanding his inner door student possessed. Liu had, over the years, taught other inner door students. Many but not all of those students still maintained contact with him. Those that did not keep in contact with him missed out on valuable information. To acknowledge his loyalty, Liu had taken Wei Ken De to the next level of training. He was pleased with the other man's intelligent questions. Liu had patiently waited for this time to come. Wei Ken De had reached a level few other students had ever reached.

Liu was now ready to take his student to the next plane of thought, understanding, and competence. This level transcended the physical and entered into what some would classify as the metaphysical. Liu knew it was a level of energy. His student was about to experience the feeling of energy many had heard about, but few had experienced.

When their discussion was over, Liu asked Wei Ken De to meditate with him. He told him that he would show him how to access specific channels of energy, which would allow him to ascend to a higher level of consciousness.

"You should feel the meridians," he told his student. "You should have some control over which meridian is receiving energy."

Softly, he told Wei Ken De to start at a specific point on a specific meridian and then will the energy to move from one acupuncture point to another and then from one meridian to another through the Connecting Meridians until he went through the Main Meridian system and the Eight Extra Meridians. Occasionally he could tell the energy had become blocked and he leaned over and gently tapped a point on Wei Ken De's body and the energy would continue on its course. He knew what the man was feeling: it was like being in heaven surrounded by pure ecstasy.

Once the meridians were open and the energy was flowing, Liu touched acupuncture points on Wei Ken De's body to further raise the energy. Sometimes he would touch only one point and sometimes it was a combination of points. The knowledge of these points came from both his own experience and the knowledge of his teachers, and now Wei Ken De possessed that knowledge. Wei Ken De would be charged with the responsibility of one day passing the knowledge on to one or two other inner door students.

Afterwards, Wei Ken De fell into a deep, meditative sleep. Liu knew that his student's body was going through a purifying process, an important thing for him to reach his full potential. His senses and innate intuition, which were critical for any martial artist, would now be heightened to where he would know what other martial artists would do before they actually did it. That was only pure energy. He would then be able to tap into his opponent's action consciousness.

"Farewell," Liu said to his sleeping student. "We will be gone when you awake, but we will meet again."

# CHAPTER TWENTY-FIVE

They had been silent most of the day and Pei Ke was beginning to get nervous. He knew they were approaching his master's home. From the events of their journey he understood at least a little of what might be waiting for them on their arrival. He had many questions, but he wisely remained silent.

"Pei Ke," Liu said later in the afternoon. "Tonight we will stay with an old family friend. I have not seen him in a number of years, but he and I played together as children. He is almost like one of the family and my brother's children would refer to him affectionately as Uncle Wu. If something is indeed wrong, he will know. He lives a short distance north of the village. I don't want anyone in the village to know that we are here, so we will skirt around it and go directly to his house."

Pei Ke tried to imagine what his master was thinking or feeling. There was no clear dent in his usual façade of calmness, but when he and Pei Ke practiced in the morning, the master seemed slower than usual, perhaps a little distracted. Pei Ke himself had been distracted as well.

He had been exhausted after his conversation with Wei Ken De, as though he had run up a mountain, but he was still unable to keep Mei Li from entering his thoughts. It was as though she had somehow left an image of her inside his eyes. Even in his fear of the upcoming events, he saw her, smiling at him and moving gracefully beside him.

Later as the sun was setting Liu and Pei Ke came over a small rise. In the distance they saw a beautiful compound surrounded by trees and shrubs. From their elevation, Pei Ke could see three buildings within the walls. To the south, he could see the outline of the village.

As they approached the front of the compound, he saw two massive doors guarding the entrance. The carvings on the doors were extremely ornate. It was obvious someone of influence resided behind the doors.

They were no closer than thirty feet from the entrance when an armed guard suddenly approached from the right side. Pei Ke was startled at the first sight of the guard. He could not tell where the man had come from. It was as though he materialized from nowhere blocking the entrance. A sword hung from his side and Pei Ke had no doubt that he knew how to use it.

Liu stopped.

"My name is Liu Bin and I would like to speak with Wu Shiang Ming."

The guard stared at both of them for a moment. He then bowed slightly indicating recognition of the name. He hurried to the door and tapped on one of its broad panels. A small portal opened and the guard whispered to someone behind the door.

The guard stood awkwardly looking at the ground and at Liu at the same time. Pei Ke thought it was clear the man knew something. If his bearing was any clue, what the man knew was not good. Liu's face was impassive as he stood, rooted to the ground.

When the doors finally opened, a girl a little younger than Pei Ke came out and ran towards Liu. She was as beautiful as Mei Li.

"Liu Bin, you have come," the girl sobbed, throwing her arms around Liu.

Liu at first was startled to see the young girl he had only seen once when she was very young. She was now a woman. He put his arms around her and held her close. Tears rolled down her cheeks as she buried one side of her face into his robe. She started to shake as she sobbed almost uncontrollably. Liu hugged her tightly. He glanced at his student and saw Pei Ke's confusion.

"Her name is Hua Yee," he said softly.

Pei Ke nodded, looking at both of them. Obviously, she had suffered some extensive ordeal. The extent of her grief told him that she alone was not the reason for the letter his master had received. Again he looked to Liu's face and for the first time, saw some emotion in Liu.

"Uncle Wu said you would come," the girl said, "and we have been waiting for you for over two weeks."

"We?" said Liu.

"She and the children," a man said from the doorway.

Liu looked up to see Wu briskly walking towards him with both arms outstretched. He encircled his arms around Liu and Hua Yee. Pei Ke saw tears in his eyes.

"You received my note," said Wu.

"No" Liu said, absently stroking Hua Yee's hair. "I received a note but it was not from you. I do not know who it was from. It only indicated that I needed to return home. I left as soon as I got it and have been traveling for almost three weeks with my student, Pei Ke. "He nodded in Pei Ke's direction.

Pei Ke bowed low to Wu, but the response was engulfed by a flurry of words from the girl.

"Uncle Bin, I did the best that I could," she said. "I followed Mother's directions and stayed in the hiding place for two days before it became intolerable. There was no place to go to the bathroom and the children were becoming restless and anxious."

Liu looked at Wu for an explanation and the other man took a deep breath.

"I'm afraid your brothers and their wives, and your nephews and nieces are all dead," he said. "The compound was attacked and they slaughtered everyone. Hua Yee and a few children, escaped only because someone had the sense to hide them." His voice caught as he spoke, but he pressed on boldly.

"I am sorry, my old friend. Let's go inside and I will tell you what I know. The children are inside waiting for you."

Pei Ke felt like he was going to be sick. He stared at Wu, then at Liu. He had spent many hours during their journey trying to imagine why Liu had been summoned home, but he had not expected this. He looked to Liu for guidance in how to react to such horrific news. The master just stood there with nothing but a tightening of his lips to suppress his own grief.

"Yes," Liu said.

Just before he entered Wu's home Liu sensed that an evilness had entered into the area. He turned abruptly to look back toward the rise in the road. He thought he saw movement in the distance, but could not be sure. He did not have to see them to know they were still there. The mysterious aggression against him during his journey began to make more sense. If they had killed his family, it made sense they would try to kill him as well.

When they were inside, Liu met for the first time some of his extended family. He chastised himself for being away for so many years. He had truly missed seeing these children grow up. Tea was brought for everyone as they sat down at the table.

"Hua Yee, you are the oldest, tell me what has happened," Liu said.

"I don't know for sure," Hua Yee said as tears once again gathered in her eyes. "It was all so sudden. I remember Mother waking me in the middle of the night. She took an amulet from around her neck and put it around my neck and told me to go hide. She said the amulet was for good luck."

Hua Yee pulled out the amulet that was tied to an old leather string and showed it to Liu Bin. Pei Ke immediately felt for the amulet that he had around his neck. They appeared to be the same. Liu looked at the amulet and nodded for her to continue.

"As mother instructed, I took the children and a basket she had given me into the underground hiding place and stayed there. When the men attacked, I heard loud voices, like people arguing, but it was in a dialect I'd never heard before, so I couldn't understand what they said.

"Mother told me to leave the door to the weapon room open, but I think she meant it as a trick to draw them away. She also gave me all these instructions about the basket, and about another, bigger basket I found in the room outside the hiding place. When the children were in the tunnel, I pushed over the bigger basket and then crawled into the tunnel and slammed shut the stone that hid the tunnel, just like she'd told me. We were all so scared, but I did my best to comfort them and to keep them quiet. It was almost impossible.

"It seems like we were hiding forever. Finally, I thought I heard father and I crawled back up the tunnel and listened at the door. I heard three distinct voices. I assumed it was the men sent by my parents to come and get us. Just as I was going to push the stone, I heard screams and what sounded like fighting. I hurried back to the children and huddled them together, trying to comfort them. I was not sure how long we'd been in there, but we had all slept twice, so I thought it must have been two days. The other children were crying and hungry and I decided we had to leave."

She looked at Wu.

"I decided to come here to Uncle Wu's, if we could not find Mother or Father. When I pushed open the stone, I saw two men lying on the ground. At first, I thought they were asleep and I froze, but I quickly realized they were dead. I couldn't tell what had killed them, until one of the children saw the snakes." She shuddered.

"They were cobras, big ones, coiled up in the closet of that room. Oh, Uncle Bin, it was all so frightening."

"It is all over now," Liu said. He put his hand on hers to comfort her and to encourage her to talk.

"The ladder was broken and there was no way for us to climb out. We called and yelled for many hours until Uncle Wu found us."

"We found them on the third day," Wu said. "And what we found was horrifying. The only reason we suspected something was wrong was that one of the outsiders came to the village to get some vegetables and he had some blood on the back of his clothes." Wu put his face in his hands before continuing.

"We don't often have strangers come to this village and when they do, the locals usually notice them. Since I am one of the local authorities, I was notified and I followed the man to his camp. They were living just two miles from your parents' compound!

"When I approached their hiding place in the forest, I overheard a conversation between the probable leader of the group and what appeared to be one of the children of your brother's servant. The child was quite young and didn't seem to know much. They kept asking him about treasure. Naturally, he knew nothing. I think they are still holding him as a hostage. He is not much value as a hostage, since he is only the son of a servant."

Liu shifted in his seat. The tea Wu's servant had brought him grew cold in his hands.

"I also heard them discussing how they killed your family. They clearly took pleasure in what they did. They were angry that they could not find any treasure or anyone of value to hold as a ransom. Your family must have put up a brave fight. I got the impression that some of the attackers were killed."

"How many men were there?" Liu asked.

Wu lifted his shoulders in anger. "I don't know exactly. Maybe ten or eleven. They had been camped there for some time and it looked as though they had been there before, during, and a short time after the attack."

Liu struggled to remain calm. He was not often forced to defend his life's decisions. He could not avoid the thought that if he had been at home, he might have prevented the massacre.

"When were you able to go to my brother's home to see what happened?"

"I went back to the village and got four men, and we went immediately to your ancestral home. The whole place had been completely torn apart. No one was alive. Even the servants were dead." He took a deep breath.

"We found your older brother and his wife and we buried them in separate graves at your ancestral burial site. The other members of your family were also buried. Actually, each person was buried in a separate grave. We marked the graves in keeping with their status. The servant and his family were buried in a separate location."

Pei Ke looked from Wu to Hua Yee to Liu, trying to find his place in this horrible tale. He was an outsider here, a meager student shunted to the margin, and though he had no desire to draw attention to himself, he felt something akin to his desire at Wei Ken De's house to comfort Mei Li. Only now, it was a desire to act, to help, to become a part of this tragedy and support his master.

He listened to all that was said and tried to process it, but his thoughts kept sticking on one point: the treasure. He knew Liu's family was wealthy, but he could not imagine a treasure large enough to warrant such a vicious attack. He wanted to be wealthy, but he couldn't imagine killing to become so.

"While we were searching the house and grounds," Wu continued, "we heard faint cries for help and discovered a movable platform in the coral. When we looked inside it was dark, but we heard children's voices and we called out."

"I heard someone calling, but I didn't know what to do," Hua Yee said. "We could not stay in the hiding place for too much longer. It smelled so bad and the children were so frightened. Nothing would comfort them. And though the snakes hadn't moved since we'd found them, we were all afraid that they would wake up and bite us." She shuddered again. Pei Ke shuddered with her. He wanted to comfort her but did not know what to do.

"We saw two men dead," Wu said, "but we didn't know how they'd died. We were startled to see the snakes when we opened the closet door. The weather had turned cold and I guess the warmest place was in the area behind that door. It was so cold that the two bodies had not decayed and the snakes were preparing to hibernate. We put the snakes in the basket and took them to the local snake handler."

"Uncle Bin, the snakes must have been in the basket that Mother told me to push over. I don't know what was in the other basket she gave me, though. She just told me to leave it, and tip the bigger basket just before I went into the tunnel."

"It was her way of keeping you safe," said Liu. "She was very wise. She knew that if there was an emergency, there would be no one to protect you, so she left the cobras in the underground storage room to be your protection. The basket you carried probably had mice in it. She did not tell you because she thought you would have been too afraid if you'd known. After the courage you have shown, however, I am not so sure."

"We took the two dead men back to the village and buried them in an unmarked grave," Wu said. "There will be no one to honor them in the future. If they have offspring, no one will come to pray at their grave site."

"Hua Yee, you are the oldest and you did well under the circumstances," said Liu.

"While we were hiding I told them the story of the Monkey King, and told them stories about you and how you went away to be a monk. I know you are not a monk, but you know what I mean: you live with the monks and lead the life of a monk." Her rambling deteriorated into tears again.

"What will happen to us now? "She rubbed the tears from her face as she looked at both Liu and Uncle Wu.

"We brought her and all the children to stay with us," said Wu.

"Arrangements will be made for you and the others," said Liu. "Do not worry,"

Liu turned to Wu and asked. "Are you sure that you only found two men?"

"Yes," said Wu.

Liu thought for a minute. He made a mental note of the discrepancy between what his niece had heard and what Wu had found.

Turning to Wu, he asked. "Did you find anything of significance when you went to the house?"

"Nothing but death and destruction."

"Do you know who did this?" Liu asked.

"No." Wu looked visibly agitated as he searched for just the right words. "It is well known that your great-grandparents made some enemies many years ago. I remember long ago there were rumors about a dispute as to the ownership of the land. The house and the surrounding property are very valuable. Maybe the outsiders wanted to take over the property?"

"It is possible, but if they wanted the land, they would still be there to claim it. Do you know where they are?"

"They have moved on, but it is not difficult to follow their tracks. It's almost as if they want to be followed by the way they leave clues."

"Has anyone gone after them?"

Wu sighed.

"No. Even though I am one of the local authorities I am in no position at my age to chase after them and arrest them. I tried to get help. The local law enforcement officer is too scared and weak to do anything. He is only really useful in carrying out the mandates of the ruling class on taxes and edicts."

Liu turned to the girl. "Hua Yee, are you sure that you do not know anything else that can help us identify these people? Do you remember anything about their conversation or dialect that would give us any clues as to their identity?"

"No, Uncle Bin. I didn't recognize the dialect they spoke."

Liu turned to Wu. "Do you know this dialect?"

"Yes. It is from the north. I don't speak it, but I can understand it. They know our dialect, though. They spoke to the servant's son, but I don't think he told them much because he is too young. He might have told them you were one of the family, but were not living at the compound. A discrete inquiry could have been all that was necessary to discover your location. Your family is the most prominent family in this area. Your lands and wealth are unmatched."

Pei Ke looked at his master and knew that their journey was not over. He looked at Hua Yee and wondered why she was not married. She was beautiful and certainly of age.

—————

Liu lay in bed that night but did not sleep. He could not calm his thoughts and raw emotions. The more he thought of the senseless killing the angrier he became. He realized his anger dominated his reason and tried desperately to concentrate on his Buddhist and Taoist training.

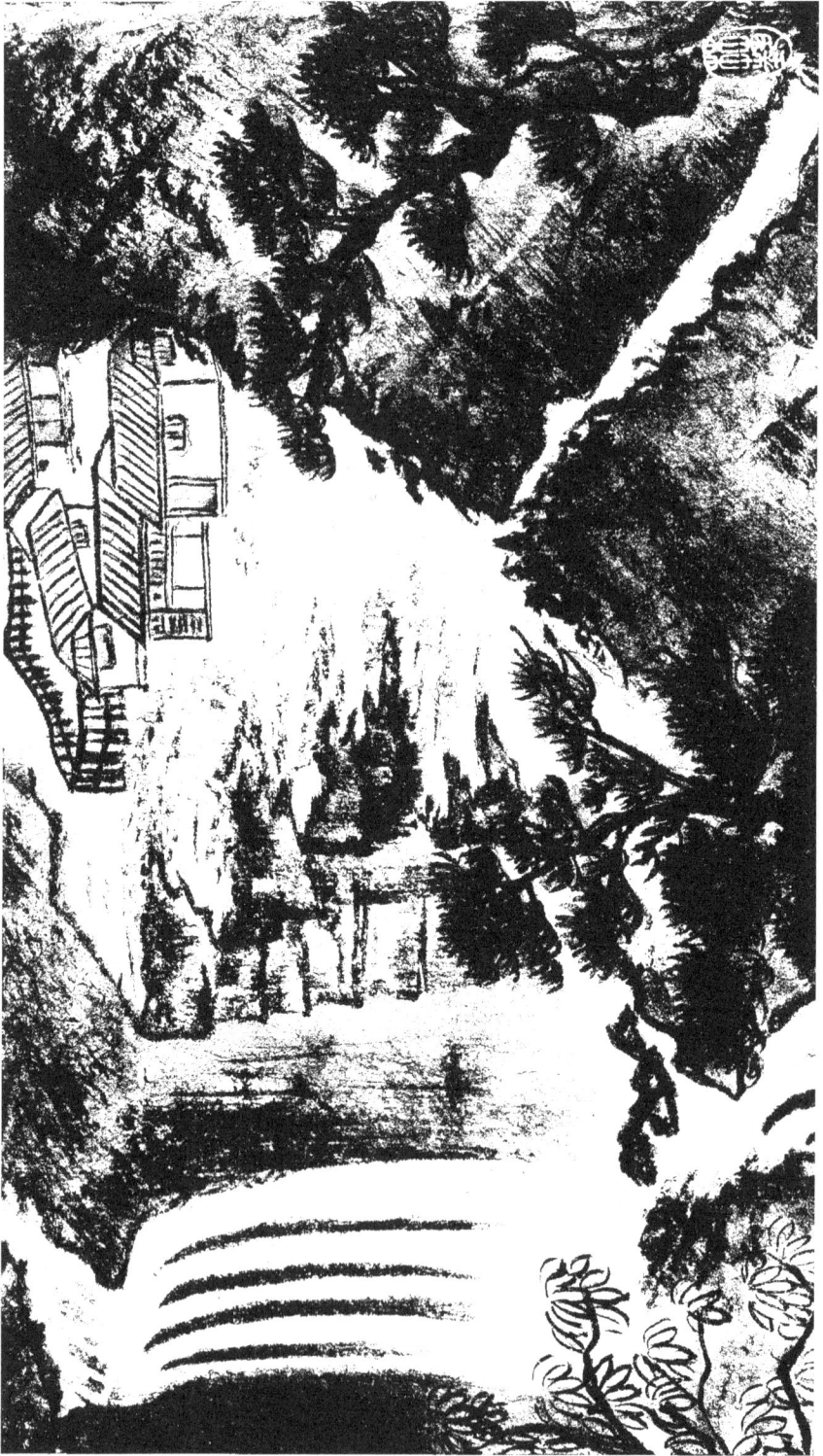

# CHAPTER TWENTY-SIX

L iu and Pei Ke left before the rising of the morning sun. The last stretch of their long—and now saddened—journey toward the Liu ancestral home took them up the side of a high mountain. This specific mountain, like many mountains, had no official name, but the Liu family had always called it the "Portal to Happiness." The road was passable, but daunting for most travelers. It was not for the faint of heart.

As they walked together, they both felt the temperature drop. Pei Ke shivered, and his breathing became labored as they neared the top of the mountain. Pei Ke turned to see if his master was all right. The pace at which they were walking would have tired most people, but Liu did not seem bothered by either the pace or the altitude. He was deeply intent on arriving at his destination.

"The snow will come shortly," Liu said. "Possibly as early as tomorrow morning or tomorrow night. Once the snow comes, unseasoned travelers cannot make it over the mountain. Many have tried and become lost when they wandered off the road."

"How far to your home?" asked Pei Ke.

"We should be there sometime today."

"Will we stay there tonight?" asked Pei Ke.

"Yes." Liu's manner indicated he would answer no more questions.

Pei Ke wondered where they would sleep and if they would be safe. Now that he knew the full story behind what had happened at Liu's ancestral home, the attacks he and his master had endured had taken on new meaning. He tried to be brave, to be a student like Wei Ken De was, but he could not ignore the iciness around his heart.

As they climbed farther up the slope, Pei Ke thought about Mei Li. He told himself that he was thinking of her to distract himself. But if he was honest with himself, he had not stopped thinking of her, except in the most terrible parts of the previous night's stories. He thought again that she would make a perfect wife for him. If only his station in life were different and he had money and a position of importance. His thoughts wandered to Hua Yee and he wished they had met under different circumstances. She too was incredibly beautiful. He wondered why she was not married. He wanted to know her better and needed to talk with her under better circumstances.

They arrived at the crest of their upward journey. The mountain's peak was still at least another day's climb, but fortunately, it was not necessary for Liu and Pei Ke to go any farther. Their present vantage point gave them a commanding view of the valley and the mountains on the far side.

The valley was even more splendid than Pei Ke had imagined from Liu's previous descriptions. He could see that every part of the valley, including its steeply sloping sides, was used to its optimum. He saw the dried rice paddies on the side of the mountain where the land had been terraced to take advantage of the downward flow of water. The tree line at this altitude gave way to areas where tea was cultivated. Rows of trees indicated orchards. A river flowed through the center of the valley. As the valley turned to the right, the river was hidden by the mountains.

Silently, Liu studied the valley, remembering how the area had looked the last time he had traveled this road. That had been a long time ago. He was pleased to see that the valley floor was unchanged. He looked off into the distance. They had to travel another fifteen minutes before they could see the houses.

"Pei Ke, this view of the valley is one of my favorites, but we are still about two hours from my home. The sun will dip behind the mountains in about four hours. Once that happens it becomes dark very fast. We must hurry so that we arrive there before nightfall. I want to see all that we can see before it gets dark."

Pei Ke risked repeating his earlier question.

"Master, will we be staying there this evening?"

Liu looked at Pei Ke for a few seconds. "I am home and want to stay here until I finished with what I need to do. When I am finished, we will go. I need to discuss plans for the estate with the local monks. Are you in a hurry to leave?"

He turned and walked down from the overlook. Pei Ke followed. As he walked, Pei Ke took in as much scenery as he could, always watching to make sure that he did not stumble or fall as the mountain slope descended rapidly. Occasionally, he looked behind him, wondering if they were still being followed, or if the danger was only before them.

Finally, as they walked around the side of the mountain, the Liu compound came into view.

———————

Both Liu and Pei Ke were deep in thought as they approached Liu's childhood home. Liu knew that normally livestock would be roaming the area, but that day the area was eerily silent and no smoke arose from the kitchen chimneys. Liu felt a coldness descend over the area as he neared the main gate.

The gate was unlocked and he pushed it open and walked into the compound. He had not walked through that gate for many years. The quiet was unsettling for both men. Liu walked slowly, observing as much as possible. Memories flooded his thoughts as he walked into the house of his older brother.

Pei Ke stayed close behind as his master went from room to room, contemplating the damage done by the attackers. As he entered his brother's bedroom, he saw the blood stains on the floor. How was it possible, he thought, for someone to enter this place and kill so many of his family? There had to be some collusion to accomplish this dastardly act.

Liu and Pei Ke walked through every building. Blood stained almost every bedroom floor. The attackers had not discriminated between adults and children; they had killed them all. It was a deliberate act to wipe out a bloodline. Liu then understood why he had been followed so closely, and why he had been attacked on his journey here. The violence would continue until whoever had done this had killed him and anyone else of the Liu bloodline that had survived.

He entered his old bedroom, where decades before he had spent many happy times. The table where he had studied so many hours was still by the window. The bed and chairs were as he had left them. The only difference was that now the floors were stained with blood. He was thankful that Wu had seen to the burials.

"Master, I am so sorry for your family."

Last night, Pei Ke had reeled at Wu's and Hua Yee's story, but now he stood in the house, looking at the blood and destruction, and he felt a deep sadness for his master.

"I remember my father telling us there was some dispute over the claims of this land, "Liu said."But he had documents signed by the emperor indicating that the land belonged to our family. He mentioned one name of a possible rival claim to the land, but he always dismissed the claim as being frivolous. Over the years, the name would occasionally come up. I will always remember the name, though I have never met any of them. However, if they killed my family, I will find them. They will not go this far and stop. There is too much for them to lose."

Pei Ke knew what his master meant by that and he looked back on all the bodies that Liu had left in his wake so far. How many men would these killers send? How many could Liu defeat?

The sun had nearly set before Liu and Pei Ke walked out of the compound and visited the family burial site some distance away. Liu and Pei Ke noted the many fresh graves and read the markers at the head of each grave. Liu bowed low in respect. Pei Ke followed and showed as much respect as was customary. Pei Ke could see tears in his master's eyes and the significance of that was not lost on him.

After a long silence, they left the cemetery and walked back to the house. Liu with tears in his eyes went directly to his older brother's house and found a lantern. He lit it as the sun dipped behind the distant mountains and cast the compound and each room into darkness.

In the main house Pei Ke followed as Liu entered what appeared to be a library. Scrolls hung on the walls and books filled the many shelves. Some of the scrolls were paintings and others were examples of perfectly executed calligraphy. Pei Ke saw the seal of his teacher on many of the scrolls. He was impressed by how scholarly the family must have been. He thought it was unusual for such a scholarly family to be so isolated.

Liu walked over to one of the walls and removed a handful of books. Most of the books were bound or tied together as was the custom of printing in those days. He reached back onto the shelf and pushed hard against the back of the wall. Pei Ke heard a click and a small portion of the wall moved forward as if someone were pushing it from behind. As the wall opened, Pei Ke saw a sword, a knife, and a small scroll jutting out from the small opening. Liu took out the document, opened the scroll, and read it quickly.

"Pei Ke, put this in the sack you are carrying. It is as important as the other things you are carrying."

"Master, what is it?"

Liu looked at Pei Ke and without a word, gave him the scroll.

Pei Ke did as he was told, wishing he had not asked the question. Liu closed the hidden alcove, leaving the knife and sword in place.

"Master, maybe we should take the sword and knife for protection. We know they are still following us."

As before, Liu did not respond and he turned away from the wall to continue his assessment of the house. The more he saw, the more he realized the human suffering that had taken place here. Evilness and hatred consumed the human mind and blinded it to all rational thinking. He agreed with what his father had always said about human nature: greed and envy sometimes led men to do things they normally would not do. Greed, envy, and hatred had driven these men to carry out this unspeakable act.

———————

That night they stayed at the compound. For Liu, it was an emotional evening. He thought of his parents and childhood and the warm family life he had experienced. His thoughts, nonetheless, always returned to the recent events. Before he finally fell asleep, he promised his father, his brothers, and all his relatives that the evilness which had destroyed the Liu family would be stopped. A resolution would be forthcoming. At first, his sleep was uneasy as he tossed and turned. Later, a calmness came over his mind and body as he meditated. In his deeply relaxed state, he willed his life energy to partially leave his body and he projected his consciousness to distant places.

Pei Ke fell asleep wondering what would happen next, but his last conscious thoughts were happily with Mei Li.

# CHAPTER TWENTY-SEVEN

Since daybreak, Liu and Pei Ke had followed the trail of the assailants. The trail led north into the mountains. As they walked Pei Ke noticed that Liu had taken the sword.

Wu was correct: the assailants were not trying to hide. It seemed as though they were leaving a trail for someone to follow. It was not a stretch to assume that they knew this person would be Liu. Only a person related to those in the compound would be interested in finding them. Liu and Pei Ke both knew it was a trap.

The temperature dropped sharply as the two men walked higher into the mountains. In a very short time, this lovely land would be covered in snow, completing the annual cycle of the land. Without the snow and spring rains, the people could not survive. They depended on the climatic changes to grow their vegetables and rice.

As they climbed farther up the slope, the lushness of the vegetation gave way to mature trees and wide spaces with no grass or vegetation. Liu knew the men he trailed were close. They needed grass for their horses.

The sun was setting as they stepped from behind a huge rock and saw guards making their rounds. Liu instantly froze in his tracks and motioned for Pei Ke to stop. They slowly ducked back behind the rock.

From his vantage point, Liu could see the whole area. It was a perfect area to camp. He saw a main tent, but he knew it was a ploy and he was not to be fooled. Whoever laid out the tents knew anyone approaching the area would have to walk uphill.

The area surrounding the back of the campsite was steep and so only three sides needed to be watched. A fire in the center of the camp illuminated the whole area as the daylight disappeared. The horses, tethered to the left and right of the tents, were facing away from the center camp area. They would give warning of anyone approaching. They had set their camp well. The only safe way to enter was from the front. To do so unobserved would require all the camp inhabitants to be asleep.

"What are we going to do?" Pei Ke asked.

Liu touched his fingers to his lips. He whispered into Pei Ke's ear. "Take this sword and wait here for me."

Liu moved away from the boulder and crept silently up the embankment toward the campsite. He would have preferred entering the camp from above, and taken the risk of sliding. The wind, however, was blowing downward and he didn't want the sound of his movements carried to the camp. The horses might detect his presence, too.

He was in no hurry. He only moved a couple of feet at a time, stopping often to watch the guards and horses.

He lingered behind a tree. From his vantage point, he saw two guards walking in a random pattern. The tree line was about fifteen feet from the guards and it was another ten feet to the campfire. Both guards would occasionally walk to the fire to warm their hands or add wood to the blaze.

The guards spoke in a northern dialect that Liu was partially familiar with. He remembered hearing the dialect when he was a child. He understood enough of the spoken words to get the context of the conversation.

He waited patiently for the camp to settle in for the night. He wanted as many men as possible to be asleep when he moved into the area. His duty this cold night brought great sorrow in his heart. Long ago, he made a vow he would now violate. He did not like the thought of what he was going to do but he had no choice. His family's blood required the action he was going to take. The evil could not remain unchecked.

Snowflakes started to fall and the men cursed their fate. Liu knew the guards would be changing soon. He planned to strike then. He waited patiently.

When the falling snow increased in intensity, the guards headed for the nearby tents. As soon as they were inside, Liu moved quietly around the periphery to the four tents in the rear of the campsite. He did not know how many men were in the camp, but by the size of the tents, he guessed that Wu was right: eight to ten. The smallest tent would probably house the servant's boy, the hostage they had taken from his brother's ancestral home. There was likely someone guarding the boy. The larger tent would hold most of the men. The leader and his most trusted guard would be in another tent. More guards would fill the last tent. Liu guessed the largest tent in the center of the campsite held the equipment they had brought with them.

He smiled grimly at the thought that they believed he would be stupid enough to fall for a trap like that. He crept to the smallest tent. The snow was falling much harder, covering up any sound he made. He thanked the gods for their help and carefully moved the peg holding down one corner of the tent. There were two people sleeping in the tent. One was much larger than the other.

Liu opened the flap of the tent and quickly straddled the larger shape. With one movement the man was dead, his neck snapped. The only sound was a slight gasp, which was only audible inside the tent. Liu threw off the covers of the smaller shape. It was the boy.

Liu put one hand over the boy's mouth and shook him gently to wake him up. The warmth of the boy's breath puffed against Liu's hand and the boy's eyes widened. The boy tried to struggle at first.

"What is your name?" asked Liu, slowly taking his hand away and indicating the need to be quiet.

"I am here to rescue you."

"Chang Song." The boy, now fully awake, started to sit up.

Liu recognized the surname of the servants who had faithfully served his family for generations.

"Do you have any clothes?"

"Only the clothes that I am wearing. My other clothes are at home."

Liu recognized the amulet around the boy's neck, which looked like a piece to a puzzle.

"Where did you get this?" he said, pointing to the amulet.

"My father gave it to me and told me I must wear it at all times. At first, one of the men wanted to take it from me. When he saw it was broken and of no value, he let me keep it. Who are you? They said no one would hurt me."

"I am not going to hurt you. My name is Liu Bin. I am the brother of Liu Ming."

"Why am I here? Where are my mother and father?"

"These men attacked the compound and killed almost everyone but you, Hua Yee, and some of the children. I will take you back, but for now, you must stay here in the tent and cover up so I know you are safe. I will come for you in a little while. The man next to you is asleep. Don't disturb him."

Liu moved the flap of the tent slightly to the left and peered outside. It was still snowing heavily. No one was around. Either the guards hadn't changed or they were not changing. He started to leave the tent, but then moved back in far enough that he could see out but not be seen. He had to wait. He turned and looked at Song. The boy was covered up totally.

Within minutes, he heard angry voices of two men who were now outside: the changing of the guard.

Minutes passed and he thought the two previous guards had settled in for the night. He peered from the tent. The new guards had their heads covered to avoid the snow. They were walking in a pattern. Liu mentally timed the pattern. He would have twenty seconds before the alarm would sound. He looked at Song, then looked out the flap at the two guards. The men were walking toward each other.

Liu intentionally relaxed the muscles in his body. With his mouth closed and his tongue touching the roof of his mouth, he concentrated on his Qi Hai acupuncture point. As he gently breathed in and out to collect the Qi, he saw the men getting closer. They would pass each other in three seconds.

He could not wait any longer. He counted out two seconds, opened the flap and quickly stood up. He ran to the closest man, covering the distance as fast as he could. Liu's right arm went forward and his hand circled the guard's throat as the guard started to struggle. Liu's other arm went to the head and around the guard's mouth as he rooted both of his feet into the earth. He inhaled through his nose. The Qi rose up through his legs into the Qi Hai point. As he exhaled through his nose, he released the collected energy in the lower part of his abdomen and with a violent snapping motion he broke the neck of the assailant. Before the guard hit the ground, Liu ran as fast as he could toward the second guard.

The second guard had reached the end of his pattern and turned around just enough to see the flash of a fist slam into his abdomen. The Hsing-Yi Chuan punch was so forceful that it knocked the wind out of him, and he buckled forward. Liu bent over, grabbed the guard's neck with both hands and squeezed tight. With a quick upward and twisting motion, he snapped the neck. The guard died instantly.

Three down and more to go, he thought. He quickly searched the bodies and found each had a sword and a knife. The swords would be useless in close quarters, so he took the knives.

He looked around the campsite to make sure no one had seen him. Everything, including the horses, was quiet. He approached the guard tent and waited for his breathing to return to normal. He gently moved the flap covering the entrance to the darkened tent and peered inside. He saw six men at most and planned his strategy. Once again, he touched the tip of his tongue to the roof of his mouth and breathed deeply. With a knife in each hand, he quietly opened the tent flap.

The first two were easy. There was no scuffle, blood gushed from the side of each guard's neck as their carotid arteries were deeply severed. The second two woke and started to shout. They were dispatched instantly as knives were thrust deeply into their hearts. The fifth one managed to pull his knife and take a stab at Liu. Liu moved swiftly to one side and blocked the thrust. He grabbed the knife hand, twisted it and broke the wrist of the guard. With another swift motion, the fifth man was dead. The sixth man ran out of the tent screaming.

Liu stepped over the bodies and followed him outside. The snow was accumulating on the ground. He saw footsteps leading from the tent toward the edge of the campsite. Two men with their swords drawn were coming toward him from another direction.

"Who are you?" the older one yelled.

"I am Liu Bin. Who are you?"

"I am Chen Su, the rightful owner of the lands and treasure taken from my great ancestors."

"You killed my brother and his family?"

"Yes, and unless you tell me where the treasure is, I am going to kill you too."

Chen Su and the other man, who looked very much like the leader that he was likely his son, charged toward Liu, their swords ready for battle. As they drew closer, they separated. The more they separated the easier it was for Liu. A swordsman needs room and two men with their swords needed to be far apart to use their weapons effectively. For Liu it was ideal. He needed only to worry about one at a time once the fight started.

The older Chen had done the talking. Liu knew that the son, who was taller and heavier, would attack first. Liu kept watching the senior Chen, but kept the son in his peripheral vision. He knew from his training and experience that he could react faster with peripheral vision than with a direct line of sight.

The instant Chen's son moved, Liu turned and moved to close the distance between them. This caught the son off guard. He was still bringing his sword to a ready position to swing at Liu when Liu grabbed the attacking arm and locked it out, then broke it as he took the sword away.

Liu turned and swung the sword without looking and sliced deeply into the son's arm. Blood squirted from the wound and the man screamed. He fell to the ground, holding his right arm, which was broken and bleeding.

Liu then swung around to face Chen.

"You are going to die, Liu," said the elder Chen.

"Your evilness will not get past this evening," said Liu as he stood up straight and pointed the sword tip toward the ground.

Old Chen stepped forward and swung his sword toward Liu's left side. Liu raised his sword to block and in one continuous motion, he swung the sword in an arc that came down on the side of Chen's neck, severing his head from his body.

"Liu Bin, he is getting away!" screamed Song.

Liu glanced at the servant boy by the tent and saw that he was right. The younger Chen was gone. He then heard the sound of a horse galloping off to the left.

Liu sighed and went to Song.

"Are you all right?"

"Yes."

"Let's go."

"Where are we going? What will happen to me?"

"You will be well cared for. Do not worry."

Liu turned and motioned for the boy to walk by his side. As they walked out of the campsite, Liu saw tears running down the boy's face. The boy turned to Liu. "Are they all dead?"

Liu looked at the boy. "They will sleep for a long time."

"What makes them sleep for so long?"

"They have no more Qi."

"Master Liu"

"Yes"

"You look very sad."

"We are both sad. You have lost your parents and I have lost my family." To himself, he added, "And I have now violated a very important tenet that I held dear."

Liu put his arm around Song's shoulders and they walked from the campsite and down the mountain side. The flickering fire of the campsite threw off enough light for him to see one person standing over another one lying on the ground.

"Pei Ke," he said softly.

He motioned for Song to stay still and silently moved forward until he could see Pei Ke standing over the body of the one guard who had escaped. The student was covered in blood and had a wild look in his eyes. Motioning for Song to follow, they walked to where Pei Ke was standing.

"We surprised each other," Pei Ke said. "I heard him coming and thought it was you, so I stepped out to greet you. He was running very fast and when he tried to stop, he slipped and crashed into me. I must have been holding the sword with the point down, because as I crumpled on top of him, the sword impaled him."

Liu was saddened that another life had been taken, but deep within himself he felt that the revenge for his family's death had been almost satisfied. He would never be able to follow Chen's son through the forest and mountains at this time of year. He wondered if and when they would meet again.

Pei Ke looked down at the man he had killed and felt guilty. He had had no desire to take a human life, and yet, he felt as though he had, in his own small way, managed to assist his master in his gruesome task. He made a promise to himself that it was the last time he would take a life. In the future, he would only heal.

The clouds moved off to the east, revealing bright moonlight as the two men and the boy walked down the mountain to Liu's home where they would stay the night.

# CHAPTER TWENTY-EIGHT

Liu, Pei Ke, and Song stayed the night at Liu's ancestral home. In the morning Liu took Chang Song to the gravesite. Once again, Liu paid respect to his grandparents, parents, and those killed in the attack.

Liu pointed out to Song where Song's parents and grandparents were buried and helped him pay proper respect to the ancestors. Liu saw the tears in the boy's eyes and they cried together.

Liu thought of his parents and the wonderful childhood he had had. As he looked at their graves, he told them he had done his duty as a filial son. He promised his brother that Hua Yee and the others would be taken care of for the rest of their lives. The ancestral lands and house were intact and his brother's death was not in vain. He told his father that he still carried the treasure with him, and the treasure at the temple would be handled according to his wishes.

Liu helped Song gather his meager belongings and they walked toward Wu Shaing Ming's house. At the crest of the mountain, Liu sat on a boulder, looking back at his ancestral home. In a loud voice he told his parents he would return one day to again pay respect. With tears in his eyes, he held on to Song's hand, turned, and continued their walk to Wu's house. Pei Ke trailed behind sadly.

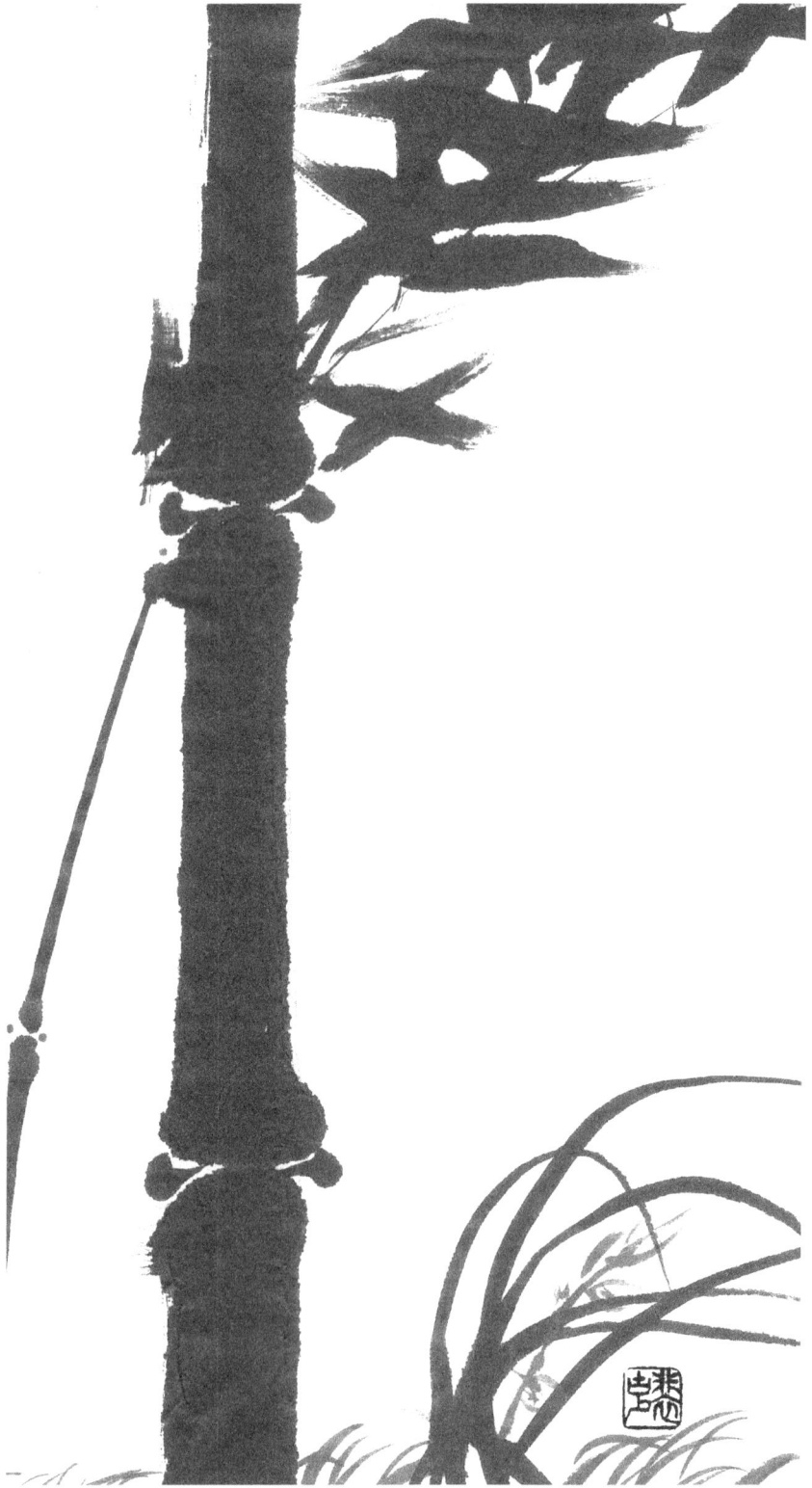

# CHAPTER TWENTY-NINE

For the next two weeks, Liu's time was spent between his ancestral home and Uncle Wu's. He talked with Hua Yee and the children and tried to explain to them in the best terms possible what had happened. He received visitors from families that wanted to offer their condolences and to once again see Liu Bin. Many questions were asked about the fate of the children and the property. Liu gave no indication to anyone what he intended to do.

After the third week, Liu went to the local Buddhist temple. The Liu family had established the temple and had been its main benefactors since its inception.

"I trust that you have taken care of matters with your family?" asked the Abbot.

Liu looked at the Abbot for a moment. "Yes. I have visited the compound daily and ensured due respect has been given to my family, especially my parents and grandparents. I made arrangements for the compound and lands to be cleaned and cared for until I decide what to do with the land, or until the young ones come of age. Hua Yee is of age to have a husband. I entrusted all this with a close family friend. I am sure you know and respect Wu Shiang Ming?"

"Of course. He is one of the elders in the village. You made a wise decision. He is also a contributor to the temple. His contributions are not quite to the extent of your father and grandfather, but nevertheless he is an important figure."

"I have asked him to discuss some personal matters with you. He will be here in a few days."

"What will you do now? If you like, arrangements can be made for you to stay at this temple for as long as you wish. Your family has been so generous to us that there is no way we can ever repay you. It would indeed be an honor for us to have you stay."

"Thank you for your generosity. I have consulted the I-Ching numerous times since I have been home. Each time, the I-Ching pointed me in the same direction. I am going to visit some friends that I have not seen in quite some time. We trained together in martial arts for many years and it would seem appropriate for me to visit with them.

"There is a matter, however, I would like to discuss with you now. It concerns a portion of the treasure belonging to my family. You are aware of what I am talking about?"

"Of course. Your father and later your elder brother and I have had more than one conversation concerning both the land holdings and the other items of wealth. As you know, some of that wealth is hidden here at the temple. Only a few of us are aware of where it is hidden. The secret has been guarded by us and will continue to be guarded."

"I am aware of the details," Liu said, "and I can assure you that I have no immediate interest in any of it. I only want to make sure that whoever gets the treasure is entitled to receive it."

"The instructions we have in writing are clear and there is no room for misinterpretation."

"Yes, I know. I was given a copy of those instructions including the location of the hiding place in the temple."

The Abbot looked at Liu for a minute. Liu sensed the man's doubt. Liu knew strict rules had been put in place to protect the treasure, and so he offered the Abbot the password to show the truth of what he had said: "Kuan Yin is one of the most adored deities in the temple and we pray at her feet."

Slowly, the Abbot nodded.

"And four pieces make a circle," Liu said. "That circle may be presented to you shortly, but I would like now to humbly ask an important favor," Liu said.

"What can we do for you? We can only offer you a place to stay." He moved about nervously as if he were afraid what Liu might ask.

"It is not for me, nor is it for my remaining family, but for Chang Song, the son of the servants. Would you take him into the temple and care for him until he comes of age? His parents were our servants and they have been loyal for so long, it seems only the right thing to do. Teach him all that you can, including the foundation of martial arts. I will compensate you for his care. Wu Shiang will make the necessary donation to the temple. At a later date I, or someone else, will check on his progress."

"It will be done as you wish," said the Abbot.

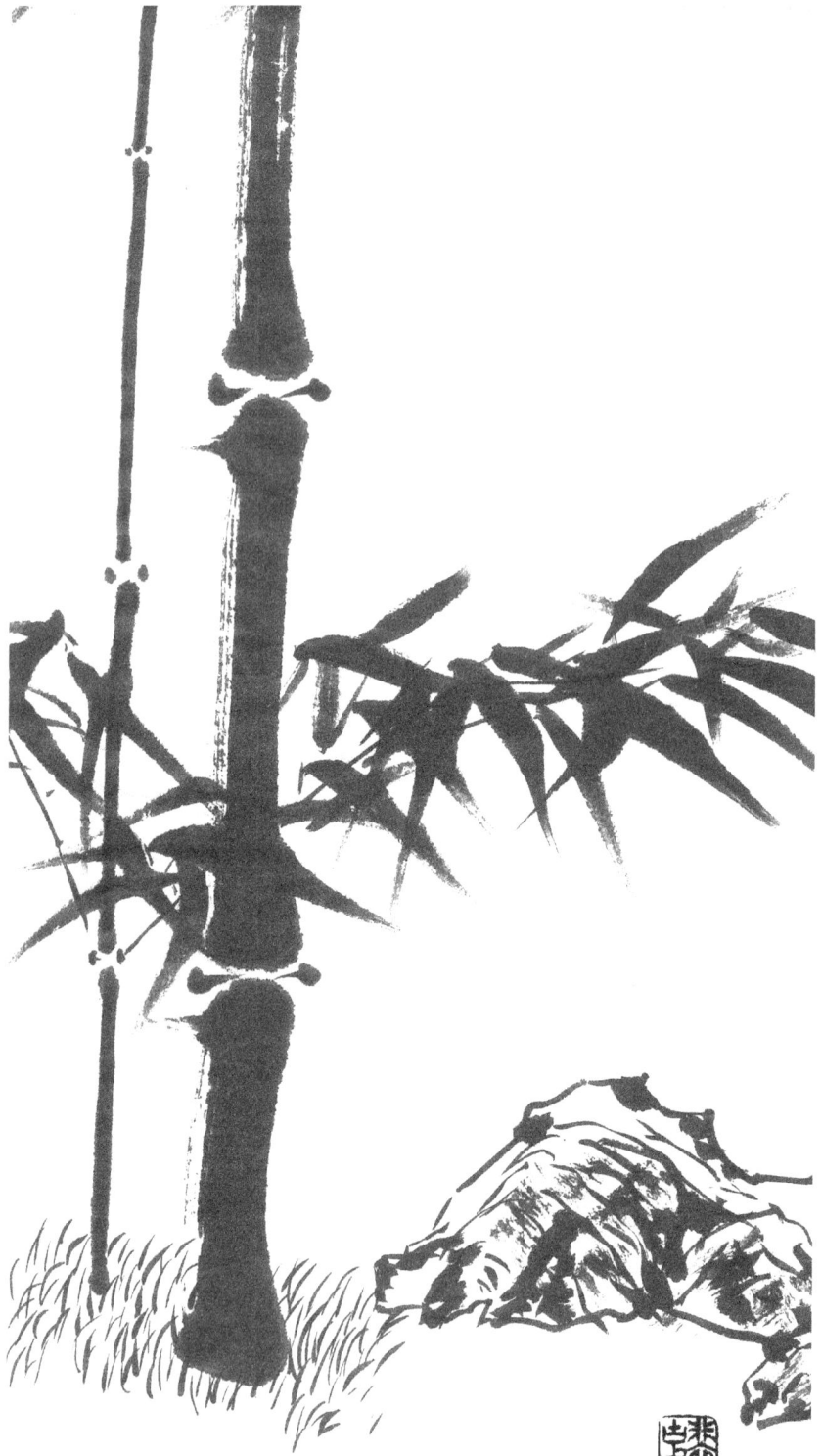

# CHAPTER THIRTY

The sun was rising in the sky as they walked from Wu Shaing Ming's home to the temple. Pei Ke tried a couple of times to engage Liu in a conversation, but Liu was deep in thought. As they approached the temple, the master turned to the student.

"Pei Ke, please let me have the sack you have been carrying for me."

"Yes, Master," said Pei Ke as he untied the straps of the large leather sack he was carrying on his back. "You have insisted I carry it this whole journey, which I have done. I cannot imagine what is in it, but it must be valuable."

He carefully handed the sack to Liu.

"Yes, Pei Ke, the contents are priceless. They are part of my family's treasures, plus the knowledge I have accumulated over these many years. What I have taught you thus far is a small part of what is written in these scrolls, and what you must learn to be a doctor, martial artist, painter, and calligrapher. This treasure of knowledge is a summation of thousands of years of Chinese medicine, including Buddhist and Taoist concepts for longevity that have been kept secret for generations. Only a handful of people possess this knowledge. Having this knowledge would enable one to live far past the normal years. It is one of the reasons I have lived so long." Liu put the sack on his back and adjusted the straps.

Pei Ke looked at his master and understood the significance of Liu's action.

"Master, what am I supposed to do now?"

"Go to the Abbot and show him the amulet you are wearing around your neck. He will tell you what to do."

"What are you going to do? I want to go with you."

"Do as I ask," said Liu.

He touched Pei Ke's arm then turned and walked away from the temple. Pei Ke stared at him. He felt a deep uncertainty inside. At the temple steps, he stopped and watched Liu walking farther and farther into the rising sun.

"Where is Teacher going and why am I here?" he said aloud. "What am I supposed to do now?"

Sadly, he entered the front door of the temple.

"Master Liu has sent me here to see the Abbot," said Pei Ke to the first monk he saw.

"Does the Abbot know you are coming?"

"I think so," said Pei Ke. "Master Liu Bin told me to come to the temple and speak with the Abbot."

"Follow me."

Pei Ke was taken to the main courtyard of the temple where he waited for a long time. The courtyard was beautiful. In fact, the temple was probably the most picturesque temple he had ever seen. When the Abbot arrived, he did not speak but motioned for Pei Ke to follow him. They walked in silence to the main altar where the statue of Kuan Yin the Goddess of Mercy was placed for all to see. Pei Ke looked at the other statues around the temple, but knew from what his parents told him that Kuan Yin was dear to the hearts of many.

"Pei Ke."

"Yes, Abbot?"

"Do you know the story of Kuan Yin?"

"Of course. She is the Goddess of Mercy. My mother always told me to go to the temple to pay respect to her."

"What else did your mother tell you about the goddess Kuan Yin?'

"That Kuan Yin listens to our prayers when we need help, and we should feel comfortable when we pray to her."

"Did Master Liu mention anything special about Kuan Yin or this spot?"

"No."

The Abbot realized that Pei Ke did not know anything about the location of the Liu treasure.

"Have you ever been in other temples?"

"Yes."

"Did you notice there is always a special place in the temple for the statue of Kuan Yin?"

"I have always noticed that her statue was there, but now that you mention it, there always is a unique place for her. In fact, my mother had a statue of Kuan Yin on an altar in our home. She would light incense, kneel, and bow many times, very fervently. Almost every home I have visited has a statue of the Goddess of Mercy."

"At any time there is sorrow, she listens to the prayers," the Abbot said. "She is always depicted with a peacefulness and a gentle radiance. Actually the story of Kuan Yin dates back many generations. Have you noticed that many of the other statues do not give you the feeling of inner peace?"

Pei Ke scanned the various statues that represented a diversity of gods.

"Yes, I have."

"Pei Ke, look over to your right. Do you see those three statues next to each other?"

"Yes."

"Do you know what they represent?"

"No."

"They are usually placed together and represent the three Star Deities. The first one is the deity Shou. You can recognize him by his high forehead. He usually carries a peach in one hand and represents health and longevity. The second Star Deity is Lu. He is the god of rank and influence. He is often seen holding a scepter. The third deity is Fu who represents happiness and wealth. He is the tallest of the three and is usually placed in the middle. Of the three which one is the most important?"

Pei Ke thought for a moment and knew that the Star Deity Fu was the most important for him, but suspected it would be the wrong answer.

"They are all important," said Pei Ke

The monk smiled knowing full well that Pei Ke had a preference.

Pei Ke noticed another, rather brightly colored statue. The color initially attracted his attention, but it was the design of the statue that prompted him to ask a question.

"Is that statue a representation of the God of the Kitchen? My mother had a statue like that."

"Yes, that is the Kitchen God. Many families worship him at the new and full moon. His statue is probably in every home. He is as important as Kuan Yin, but for a different reason."

"That painting of bamboo on the wall next to the statue of Kuan Yin is beautiful," said Pei Ke.

"Did your parents teach you how to read?" The monk looked intently at Pei Ke.

"Yes, my parents taught me a little."

"Go to the scroll and read the characters."

Pei Ke walked across the hall to the painting, confused. So far, the Abbot had said nothing about Master Liu or why he had been sent here. As he got closer to the scroll, he could make out the characters. They were written in excellent penmanship. As he read each character, he gasped as he recognized the calligraphy of Master Liu and saw his seal. He turned to the monk and the monk nodded.

"How exceptional to have such beautiful writing!" said Pei Ke. "Master Liu can do so many things and he does each one so well. There must be something he has that others do not have. He truly blends with the Tao. He is always peaceful, patient, and happy. If I could be a small part of what he is, I would be happy. Of course, everything has a price. I do not know if I could do everything he has done to get where he is now."

"Why have you come to see me?" asked the Abbot.

"Master Liu sent me to see you and to let you look at this amulet. I have been wearing it for some time now. Master gave it to me when we left the temple on our journey to his ancestral home. He said you would instruct me on what to do next."

"Yes, I spoke with Master Liu. Do you know who he is?"

"Yes, he is my teacher."

He walked closer to Pei Ke.

"Let me see the amulet," said the Abbot, holding out his hand.

The Abbot looked at the amulet for a long time. Then he stared at Pei Ke, who instinctively knew the monk was looking into his soul. A shudder went through his body as the Abbot continued his stare.

"Wait here." The Abbot cradled the amulet in his hand and walked toward an archway that led into a long hallway. "You may look, but do not touch anything."

Pei Ke gazed at the beautiful statues and paintings. Energy seemed to flow through the temple, going from one statue to another. It was as if each statue enhanced the energy of the other statues, so that the total sum of their energy was greater than the sum of each individual statue. It reminded Pei Ke of the interconnectedness of the Tao, where the harmony of all things is sought. His thoughts turned to Liu Bin. Why had Master Liu told him to come here and where had he gone? Mixed feelings of happiness and sorrow came over him. The events of the last month had been exhausting and confusing and he felt his emotions frayed and fragile.

"Pei Ke."

The voice startled Pei Ke. He quickly turned to see a tall monk dressed in a long, flowing robe holding on to a scroll. No one had been there a moment ago.

"I am Master Chan. The Abbot gave me Master Liu's amulet and sent me to talk with you. You don't understand, but a great mystery has been solved today. "He held up a hand to forestall any of Pei Ke's questions.

"Before I explain, I will tell you more about the Liu family and this temple. Master Liu's grandfather and father were instrumental in the initial design and building of this temple. His father's generosity was what made this temple successful. Many years ago, Liu's father feared that the family treasure would be stolen or squandered, so he decided to put his wealth here in the temple for safekeeping.

"He fashioned a large amulet that looked like a coin and could be separated into four pieces. Each piece of the coin or amulet had a small hole near the edge so a string could be put through the hole. The amulet was meant to be worn around the neck. He gave one piece to his faithful servant and the servant's family for all their years of service. One piece went to the eldest son. The third piece went to the Abbot of this temple. The fourth piece went to Master Liu. The father judged correctly that Liu would have no interest in the money or earthly goods, but would make sure his wishes were carried out.

"The instructions that are written on this scroll leave no room for interpretation. When the Abbot has all four amulets in his possession, he is to distribute the treasure equally to those who have presented the amulet pieces. The only possible reason the pieces would be brought to the temple was because of a calamity within the family.

"With the deaths of most of the Liu family and the young ages of the remaining children, it is an appropriate time to have the pieces of this amulet brought to the temple. If there is the slightest doubt as to the correct owner or how the amulet was acquired, that portion of the fortune would go to the poor. No one person can receive more than one fourth of the treasure."

"What does this have to do with me?" Pei Ke said, "I am not part of the Liu family."

"You are in possession of one piece of the original amulet. You have acquired it legitimately. We have accounted for the other three pieces. The servant's son has one piece, Hua Yee has another, you have one, and of course the temple has one. The temple will hold two fourths of the treasure because the last remaining heir to the servant's family will live here until he is of age. Then, he will receive his rightful portion. As decreed, the temple receives one fourth. The eldest of the Liu family, other than Master Liu, is Hua Yee.

"Traditionally, the treasure should go to the eldest son, but at Master Liu's personal instructions, the third part of the fortune will pass to Hua Yee and the other children, who will live with Mr. Wu. When they come of age, arrangements will be made for them by either Liu Bin or Wu. The last part goes to you. The title to the land will remain with Master Liu and looked after by Mr. Wu."

Pei Ke was stunned by the monk's words. "What? Why me?" He paused for a moment. "Did Master Liu tell you where he is going?"

"Master Liu has asked us to give you a choice. You may take your part of the treasure and his good wishes, or you may continue as his student, leaving the treasure to the poor."

Pei Ke looked in the direction he had last seen Liu. He turned back to the monk. "Where has Master Liu gone?"

"Master Liu will spend his remaining years furthering his spiritual enlightenment."

"Did he tell you where he was going?"

"Yes, I know where Master Liu is initially headed, but I am not at liberty to tell you at this time. You must choose to do what you think is best for you. Master Liu has no use for such worldly treasures in his travels."

"What will the temple do with Master Liu's fourth of the treasure?"

"I am not permitted to discuss temple matters with you."

Tears formed in Pei Ke's eyes as he looked at the monk and then back to the path Liu had taken. He again thought of Wei Ken De's daughter, Mei Li. She was undoubtedly the most beautiful woman he had ever met and he was sure she liked him. He thought of Hua Yee and her sorrow. She also was strikingly beautiful. Either one would make a perfect wife.

"I have always been poor," he said to the monk. "My whole family has been poor. I was raised poor. I have always dreamed of having money and enjoying the comforts and status of the wealthy. What should I do? What is the treasure?"

The monk shook his head.

"I cannot make a decision for you, nor can I give you any details about the treasure, but I can tell you this treasure will fulfill your physical and spiritual needs beyond all your dreams. Many have searched unsuccessfully and have even died attempting to obtain such a treasure."

Others have killed for it, Pei Ke thought grimly. He looked up at the statue of Kuan Yin and prayed as he had never prayed before. He sought guidance, for his emotions clouded his mind. It felt as if he were in a bad dream and all he wanted was to wake up.

"You need all four pieces of the amulet at one time to get the treasure?"

"Yes," the monk said. "We need them together at one time to insure that they belong to the rightful owners. Even though there are four pieces, they fit together in a certain pattern to validate that they are the true pieces."

"When do all the amulet holders come together?"

"Now that we know who the rightful owners are, we can arrange for that to happen."

"May I have the amulet back?"

The monk, quite surprised, gave the amulet back to Pei Ke.

"Master Liu spoke with the Abbot the other day and instructed the Abbot to give you one last message," the monk said.

"What is the message," he asked.

"What is your decision?"

"Why is it so important that I make a choice now?"

"Life is a series of decisions. We make them based on the best information we have available at the time. What is your decision?"

"What happens if I don't decide and keep the amulet?"

"Nothing happens and the treasure stays where it is."

"Master Chan, it is impossible for me to decide and so I decide not to choose."

"To not make a decision is in itself a decision. Master Liu anticipated your response. Please follow me to the Abbot."

As Pei Ke complied, he thought of his relationship with Master Liu. He thought of his parents and the implications of being wealthy. He thought of both Mei Li and Hua Yee and how beautiful they were. Would it now be possible with money to have everything he always wanted, including a wife? He thought about practicing martial arts. He thought of being a doctor and treating patients.

When they arrived at the Abbot's quarters, the monk motioned Pei Ke to sit down and the monk took his leave. The Abbot looked at him for a few moments.

Pei Ke was about to ask a question when the Abbot spoke.

"Have you made a decision yet? It is important you make a decision today."

"No, I cannot. Part of me wants to take the treasure and live comfortably for the rest of my life, and part of me wants to forsake the treasure and follow Master Liu. I cannot calm my mind so that I may decide."

The Abbot rose and deliberately walked to where Pei Ke was sitting. He touched two acupuncture points on Pei Ke's head. A deep relaxation came over him. It felt as if there were a connection between these two points. Energy ran through his body and his muscles relaxed to the point of weakness. His mind calmed and became peaceful. The Abbot continued to touch acupuncture points, always in a combination of one point with another. First the hand and foot, and then wrist and ankle, and then the arm and foot, and last the elbow and the leg. He did this first on the left side of the body because Pei Ke was male and then on the right side of the body.

Once finished, the Abbot touched the spiritual points, again starting on the left side of Pei Ke's body, followed by the right side, and the feeling of relaxation became deeper. Pei Ke felt as if he were floating on a cloud. Finally, the Abbot touched the points that help people in their decision-making processes.

"You must lay down now," said the Abbot.

As Pei Ke lay down, he knew before his head touched the tea-scented pillow that when he woke up he would know his decision. His last thoughts before falling asleep were with Mei Li, Hua Yee and Master Liu.

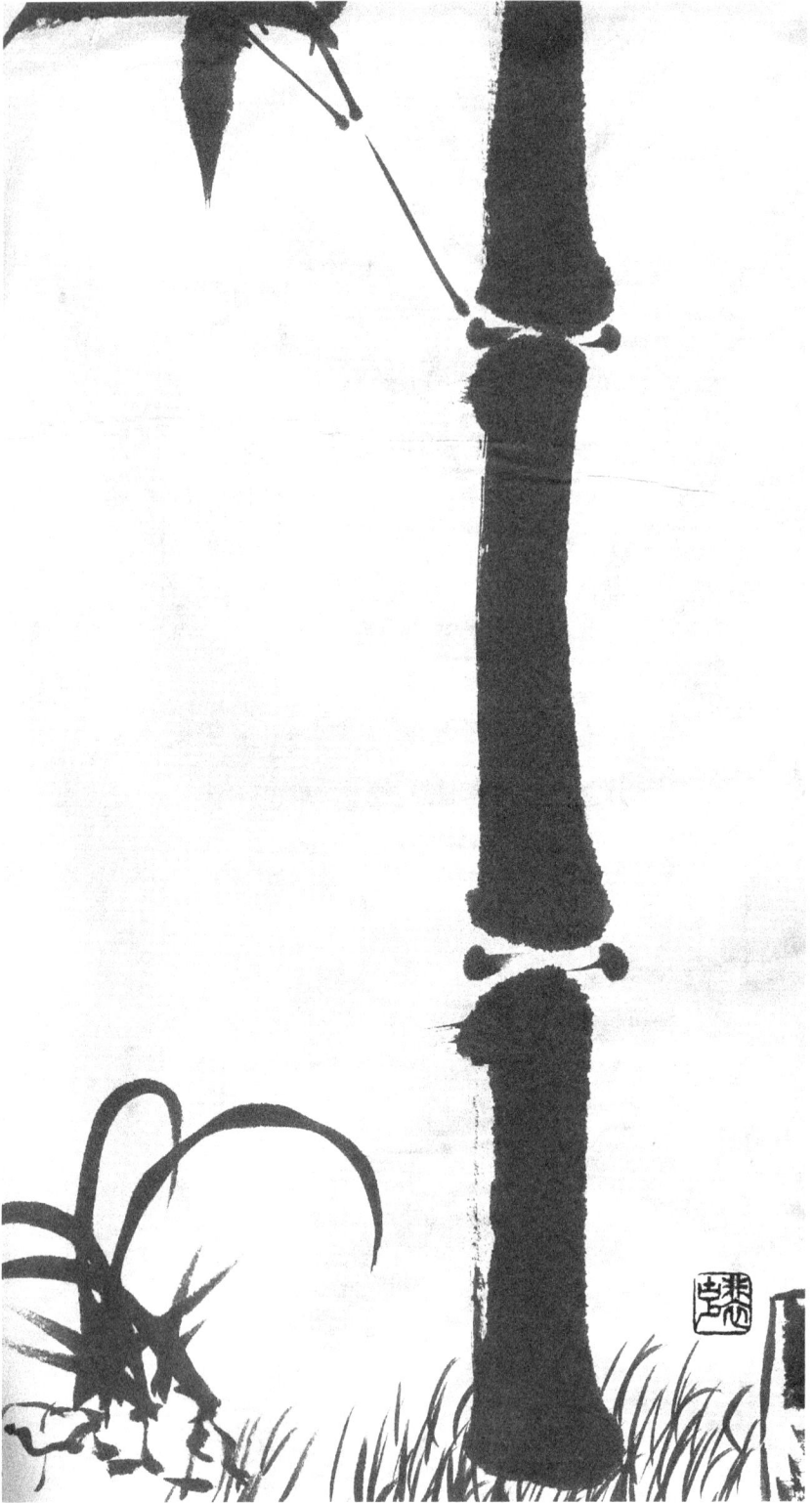

# EPILOGUE

Liu carefully balanced the sack on his back and walked on the road leading to Beijing. He had friends there within the martial arts community and he would visit them. Life in his former temple was not what he wanted at the moment. Any temple would welcome his presence, but he had other plans.

Few knew as much as Liu about martial arts, literature, philosophy, painting, poetry, calligraphy, and medicine. Some masters had more knowledge in their individual specialties, but few knew as much about so many topics. It takes a master a lifetime to be the best in any one talent. Even though he was comfortable with what he knew and where he was, he yearned for more insight into the Universal Tao.

Liu also knew the decision Pei Ke would make. Liu did not look back as he deliberately chose the road to the left when he came to the split in the road.

Few took this road for it was the more difficult way to his destination, but it afforded him the most peace. All his life he had chosen roads no one else had taken. This time was no different. In fact, he longed for the peacefulness. He was in no hurry.

The road twisted abruptly to the left and eyes again followed him. Liu sensed their presence but kept on walking. Time would be on his side. This journey was like all of his journeys. He was at peace with the Tao, and that made all the difference.

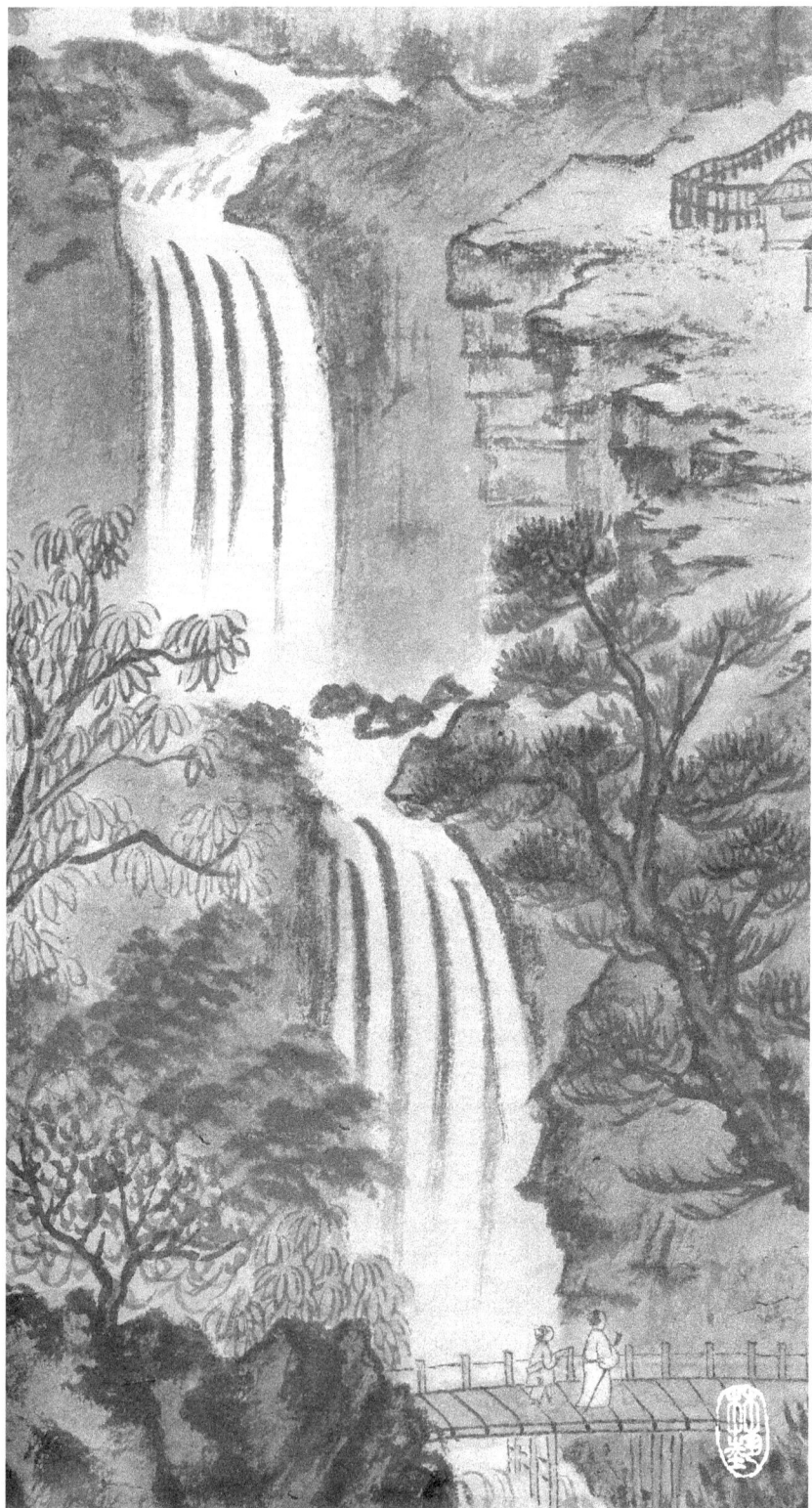

CPSIA information can be obtained
at www.ICGtesting.com
Printed in the USA
BVHW040409211218
536164BV00015B/696/P

9 781441 439208